THE STEROIDS GAME

CHARLES E. YESALIS, MPH, ScD
The Pennsylvania State University

VIRGINIA S. COWART
Cowart and Associates

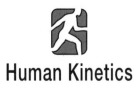

Human Kinetics

Library of Congress Cataloging-in-Publication Data

Yesalis, Charles E.
 The steroids game / by Charles E. Yesalis and Virginia S. Cowart
  p.   cm.
 Includes bibliographical references and index.
 ISBN 0-88011-494-0
 1. Anabolic steroids – Health aspects 2. Doping in sports.
I. Cowart, Virginia S., 1937- . II. Title
RC1230.Y47   1998
615'.7—dc21 --dc21
[615'.7]   97-45859
                                                                   CIP

ISBN: 0-88011-494-0

Developmental Editor: Kirby Mittlemeier; **Managing Editors:** Jacqueline Eaton Blakley,
Melinda Graham; **Copyeditor:** Heather Stith; **Proofreader:** Alesha Thompson; **Indexer:**
Joan Griffitts; **Graphic Designer:** Nancy Rasmus: **Graphic Artist:** Tara Welsch; **Photo
Editor:** Boyd La Foon; **Cover Designer:** Jack Davis; **Illustrator**: Joe Bellis and Tom
Roberts; **Printer:** United Graphics

Figure 1.1 Reprinted, by permission, from W.E. Buckley, C.E. Yesalis, K.E. Friedl, W.A.
Anderson, A.L. Strait, and J.E. Wright, 1988, "Estimated prevalence of anabolic steroid use
among male high school seniors," *Journal of the American Medical Association,* **260** (23),
pp. 3441-3445. Figure 1.2 Adapted, by permission, from W.E. Buckley, et. al., 1988
"Estimated prevalence of anabolic steroid use among male high school seniors," *Journal
of the American Medical Association,* **260** (23), pp. 3441-3445.

Human Kinetics books are available at special discounts for bulk purchase. Special editions
or book excerpts can also be created to specification. For details, contact the Special Sales
Manager at Human Kinetics.

Printed in the United States of America   10 9 8 7 6 5 4 3 2 1

Human Kinetics
Web site: http://www.humankinetics.com/

United States: Human Kinetics, P.O. Box
5076, Champaign, IL 61825-5076
1-800-747-4457
e-mail: humank@hkusa.com

Canada: Human Kinetics, Box 24040,
Windsor, ON N8Y 4Y9
1-800-465-7301 (in Canada only)
e-mail: humank@hkcanada.com

Europe: Human Kinetics, P.O. Box IW14,
Leeds LS16 6TR, United Kingdom
(44) 1132 781708
e-mail: humank@hkeurope.com

Australia: Human Kinetics, 57A Price
Avenue, Lower Mitcham, South Australia
5062
(088) 277 1555
e-mail: humank@hkaustralia.com

New Zealand: Human Kinetics, P.O. Box
105-231, Auckland 1
(09) 523 3462
e-mail: humank@hknewz.com

CONTENTS

FOREWORD

Joe Paterno
Professor and Head Football Coach
The Pennsylvania State University

Stopping steroid abuse in sports—the subject of this book—should be a major goal for all athletes, coaches, and parents. In my opinion, society still does not fully recognize the negative effects that these drugs have on the health of athletes, and on the way sports are played. There is little doubt in my mind that the use of anabolic steroids has had a substantial negative impact on collegiate football players and on the game itself. I am very concerned about the potential for physical harm to players, which may not show up until well after their football careers are over.

Medical researchers have done a good job demonstrating a number of health risks run by individual users, but the pressures to use these drugs anyway can be very strong. In some sports, athletes who don't want to use steroids often believe that they cannot be competitive. A coach who tries to maintain a clean team may be putting his players at a disadvantage when they compete against teams who are artificially bulked up with steroids.

Some coaches do not agree with me about the dangers of anabolic steroids to the individual. Others have stated that they do not believe the drugs necessarily give players an advantage. However, I think they do give players a tremendous physical advantage. It is the price of that advantage that worries me. I believe that I have seen steroids at work in the development of certain high school players. You can actually see differences in physical development and competitiveness.

It is hard for coaches to talk with athletes about the subject of steroid use, much less agree on a plan of action. At Penn State we have coached many fine young athletes, and we are concerned not only about the quality of their athletic skills but also about the quality of their lives. We get a lot of young people at Penn State who aspire to be professionals and who have already devoted years of preparation to their careers. Many of them come from families who have put tremendous pressure on them to become professional football players. I think this is true in all the top programs. Students hope to get an education, but they also want to be in a position where they can make a lot of money very early. When it became possible to earn big money in athletics, the pressure to be successful and win became much more intense. When that situation is combined with the availability of drugs that can help an athlete achieve his goals, the pressure to use the drugs is great.

How does all this affect the game of football? The notion that comes most immediately to mind is that it is hard to maintain a level playing field when some players and teams get an edge from drugs and others don't. We would like to think that drug testing would keep us out of trouble, but drug testing has not been as effective as we had hoped it would be. Users can be successful at beating the system.

We test at Penn State beyond what is required by the NCAA. I asked the NCAA to give me a list of other teams who were willing to be tested but, unfortunately, they would not give me those names. I wanted to find out if our opponents were also willing to be tested.

Even with testing, I could not tell you for sure that we do not have kids at Penn State who use steroids. My trainers talk with the players in the weight room. If a kid has put on weight, they might even ask the doctor if he thinks it's legitimate. We are concerned and try to be aware of the potential. But still, I could not unequivocally tell you we might not have some people who use them.

Personally, I think the key to stopping steroid abuse is preventing it, so there should be educational programs for young kids. Even if we continue with some form of testing, the job will be much simpler if young people develop an anti-steroid bias early in life. It isn't enough just to tell them that steroids are dangerous. We know these same young people experiment with tobacco, alcohol, and other drugs even though they know the dangers. The focus should be positive, on how kids can achieve their physical development goals without drugs. Coaches and parents should work together to make sure their athletic goals are realistic and attainable. Otherwise we risk creating an environment that encourages the use of steroids.

We also need to reinforce ethics and let athletes know that using steroids is a form of cheating and that victories achieved through drug use are hollow victories. While competition builds character, and winning is an important goal, we must make it clear to our kids that to win at the cost of your health, breaking the law, and cheating is wrong and cannot be justified.

All of us who care about sports competition must assume greater responsibility for stopping steroid abuse and making sports competition safer and fairer. find that what I will do in this paper

INTRODUCTION

In the fall of 1996, *Newsweek* magazine ran a cover story on testosterone and its effects on aging. According to the article, men who take testosterone can stave off some of the effects of getting older, including loss of muscle mass, strength, energy, and libido. What was most interesting was that the widespread use of testosterone in athletes was not mentioned at all! Yet testosterone, the primary male sex hormone, is the basis for all anabolic steroids.

Also in the fall of 1996, several news magazines featured stories about the increase in recreational drug use, heroin specifically, among youth. After a decline of several years in the use of this dangerous drug, teenagers are again experimenting. With the emphasis in recent years on anti-drug campaigns, how was it possible that anyone missed the message that heroin is a life wrecker and a killer?

How are these separate messages about different types of drug use tied together? They are associated because these articles illustrate the American ambivalence about drug taking. As a nation, we rely heavily on pills. Many people take vitamins and other so-called supplements such as creatine, DHEA, and melatonin in dosages that constitute drug treatment. It would be possible to conclude from advertising that nothing in the human body works very well and must always be assisted by medications. We fear aging and psychological distress, and we believe drugs can help.

You may be surprised to learn that Americans have been struggling with drug control problems for more than 100 years. For a brief period at the turn of the century, cocaine was even legal in the United States. At the time of the Civil War, a number of people were addicted to an opium-based preparation called laudanum that was used to treat pain and discomfort. One researcher has suggested that mood alteration is a human drive, and if that is so, it may be difficult to ever stop recreational drug use completely.

Until the advent of modern chemistry, physical alteration through drugs was not possible. That is no longer the case. For instance, children born with the genetic code for dwarfism can be treated with human growth hormones and develop normally. The sex hormones that are responsible for changing boys to men at puberty can be taken in synthetic form by adult males and females to gain strength and power; this has been happening in the athletic community for more than 40 years.

There are two important things to bear in mind about taking hormones. First, they are very powerful drugs that affect both mind and body, and we do not know what their long-term effects may be. Certainly, there are some mostly reversible short-term negative effects. Second, when elite athletes take drugs in secret to enhance their physical sports performance, they alter the whole nature of the sports contest.

The fact that these drugs are dangerous is not the only reason to bar them. Many sports carry an inherent risk of injury—look at bobsledding, skiing, football, gymnastics, and wrestling, just to name a few. However, suppose that a drug that made athletes faster was available. A cross-country skier who had invested 20 years in learning his sport would certainly be heartbroken to be beaten by a skier whose performance was improved with such a drug. Is that a fair contest? Is that what we want from sports?

Ask yourself if you care whether professional, Olympic, or even college athletes use anabolic steroids and other drugs to enhance their sports performance. In a drug-tolerant society, many people not only don't care, they don't understand why it should be a matter of public concern. Some fans reason that sports have become a combination of entertainment and big business, and the important items are good matchups, action, outstanding performances, and appealing athletes. If an athlete, especially one who is highly paid, wants to take drugs to make the magic happen, what's the difference?

Now think about what sports represents: the finest in physical development and human striving and will. Horses are drug-tested with no objections because everyone agrees that it wouldn't be a level track if some horses were doped and others were not. What would be the point of such a contest?

In 1992, the world sympathized with figure skater Nancy Kerrigan when a hired thug struck her across the knee with a steel rod to boost her rival's chances at the U.S. Figure Skating title. This was clearly unfair, but it has been hard for the public to perceive that contests where some participants take drugs to enhance their performance, and others don't, are rigged the same way the skating championship was rigged by physically knocking Kerrigan out of the competition. The difference is that we could easily see the one unfair and illegal act, whereas drug use is a hidden, secretive behavior.

Trying to get an edge on the competition is an old, old story. The legendary berserkers of Norse mythology took a hallucinogenic extract from toads for its stimulating effect. The ancient Greeks fancied hallucinogenic mushrooms and sesame seeds; gladiators at the Coliseum in Rome took natural stimulants to overcome fatigue and injury. South American Indians chewed coca leaves to increase endurance.

In the 20th century, anabolic steroids are the performance-enhancing drug of choice. Most of the athletic community accepts the fact that anabolic steroids enhance strength, muscularity, and the capacity to train, although the extent to which this occurs and under what circumstances still is not completely understood. The downside is that steroids have been linked to negative, even fatal effects in some individuals.

There are those who argue in favor of legalizing all drugs, leaving athletes and others to do as they wish. Forget drug testing, they say. In this type of climate, skater Kerrigan might have been obliged to hire her own thug to menace other competitors or to surround herself with bodyguards. If there were no constraints on the use of performance-enhancing substances, the pressure on all athletes to take these drugs would be tremendous. For instance, in bodybuilding, there have been several drug-related deaths during the past few years, and drug use is so common that non-drug-using bodybuilders can no longer compete successfully at the elite level.

Some fans *are* bothered by drug use in sport. They still see athletes as role models regardless of whether athletes want to be viewed in that light, and they see sports as a way of building character. Unfortunately, some of the fans who claim to be bothered by drug use often adopt an "ignorance is bliss" attitude, preferring to view the problem as being limited to a few scoundrels. As a consequence of public reaction, various sports organizations have spent far too much effort marketing a drug-free image, and too little effort making it a matter of fact. The fact that no positive drug tests are reported does not always mean a problem doesn't exist. This misconception has resulted in serious self-deception at the collegiate, professional, and Olympic levels.

The use of anabolic steroids and other drugs to enhance athletic performance remains the greatest problem in sports today. Moreover, it isn't just confined to professional and Olympic athletes. We have had evidence for almost a decade that high school and even junior high students are using anabolic steroids during the physically and emotionally vulnerable period when their own hormonal cycles are changing. Widespread use by younger individuals, both athletes and non-athletes, appears to be a phenomenon of the last decade. Recently the American Academy of Pediatrics concluded, "To our knowledge, no study has identified an adolescent population without the temptation and risks of anabolic steroid use. Furthermore, no study has been published showing a decrease in the prevalence of anabolic steroid use over time . . . ." (page 906). Even though our knowledge about these drugs is growing steadily, the strategies for prevention and intervention are still unfolding.

We need to educate ourselves about anabolic steroids for several very good reasons:

- An athlete may suffer physical and psychological harm because of steroids.

- The use of steroids for nonmedical purposes is a violation of state and federal laws.

- Using anabolic steroids is cheating and violates the rules of virtually every sport.

- Steroids contaminate sports because results are obtained by unnatural means.

Drug testing is not the answer by itself. Not only is testing costly, but there are loopholes that help many users beat the system. Also, there are substances for which there is, as yet, no test. The truth is when we depend solely on drug testing to protect sport, we take the responsibility for being clean away from the athletes and sports organizations.

To stop the use of steroids in sport, we must know what is really going on. How much cheating goes on and by whom? What substances are being used? What can parents of athletes do? What should coaches stress? This book has several objectives. The first is to inform readers about anabolic steroids, what they are, how they work, and their effects on health and performance. The second part of the book covers prevention measures, drug testing, laws, prevention programs, and alternatives. The third part of the book describes some of the problems that have been encountered and looks to the future.

If cheating is condoned because we don't see it happen, it still erodes the meaning of sportsmanship. If sportsmanship is lost from sports, the lesson taught by example to the young people of the United States and the world is that cheating is OK if you don't get caught. A society without ethics is in danger of becoming no society at all. That is why the question of using drugs to enhance sports performance is important to each of us.

UNDERSTANDING STEROIDS

One of the most important tools for combating steroid use is knowledge. The first four chapters of this book provide a basic framework of knowledge about these drugs, what they are, how they work, and what can be expected in terms of negative effects on health and behavior. Steroid taking is nearly always a very secret activity, hidden from public view. In the early days when use was confined mostly to elite athletes, it was customary to share information gained through personal experience, but that is no longer the case.

Moreover, although it is true that at one time steroid use was almost exclusively the province of body builders and Olympic and professional athletes in the strength and endurance sports, it has long since moved into the mainstream. The most popular public image of steroid users involves bulging muscles, superhuman strength, and a raging temper. Think of a 300 lb. professional football lineman with a 4.8 second 40-yard dash or a bodybuilder who requires professional tailoring to disguise his oversize arms, thighs, and chest. Although either of those individuals might be a steroid user, it could also be the affable trainer at the gym, your aerobics instructor, a local fireman, a dancer, or a high school kid hoping for a college scholarship.

Even though athletes have been using steroids for nearly half a century, we did not have reliable data on who the users were until the late 1980s. Since that time, several studies have established a figure of approximately 1 million past or current steroid users in the United

States. Because of these studies, we now know that more than half a million adolescents and preteens have experimented with steroids.

Because we know that younger kids are trying steroids, any intervention to stop steroid use must begin early. When the youngest users are taking drugs because of concerns with body shape and size, they are more vulnerable in every way. Many individuals long for increased strength and power. They cannot expect, of course, to get the type of gains that are seen in conditioned athletes.

The observation of a link between the male sex organs and physical strength is age-old. However, it was not until the 1930s that scientists successfully synthesized testosterone. All anabolic steroids trace their origin to the primary male sex hormone, testosterone, but there are many different chemical formulations, and the list is long and still growing. To date, no one has been able to completely divorce the masculinizing element of steroids from the tissue-building element.

A common source of information about most drugs is physicians, except in the case of anabolic steroids. Although physicians did prescribe steroids for athletes in the early days, they have not been a major source of supply for some time, both because of their knowledge about negative health effects and because steroids are now state and federally regulated drugs.

Many athletes stopped using physicians as a source of steroid information in the 1960s and '70s when a disagreement about whether steroids were effective flared up after the first steroid studies showed contradictory results. Some studies reported strength and muscle gains; others did not. The lack of agreement led many physicians to believe steroids were not effective, and this position caused them to lose credibility with the sports community. Many athletes, by that time, had experienced gains in strength and muscle for themselves by using steroids. This section explains why some scientists continued to argue the point while steroid use spread rapidly.

Unlike some European countries, the United States has never had a government-sponsored steroid research program. However, East Germany under communism was noted for its highly developed drug-aided sports programs that were developed with the cooperation of government officials, physicians, researchers, coaches, and physical trainers.

The health risks that are set out in Part I of this book can be divided into short-term and long-term dangers. Most short-term adverse effects have proven to be reversible, including sterility, changes in cholesterol levels, and acne. However, recent information suggests that a small percentage of steroid users are at immediate risk of severe heart disease and stroke. While the long-term health risk of taking steroids is unfortunately still unclear, it is naïve to believe that experimenting with such powerful drugs is without consequence. You can't fool Mother Nature. Moreover, it may be that other long-term health consequences may come to light as former steroid users age.

Too often, steroid users discount the dangers of the drugs, probably because they do not pose the same type of immediate danger as a house fire or dose of poison. Athletes haven't dropped dead on the streets or even in the locker rooms because they took steroids. However, several have died in circumstances that led most experts to conclude that their steroid use played a major role in shortening their lives.

The negative effects of steroids on behavior are a subject of some controversy. Much has been written in recent years about an association between steroid taking and violent rages. Where the absolute risk may be open to debate, most experts do agree that some individuals will have psychological problems as a result of taking steroids. It stands to reason that those who are better adjusted psychologically will have fewer consequences than those who are farther out on the behavior continuum, but nobody really knows who is at risk.

The special hazards faced by women who take steroids makes it hard to comprehend the fact that this type of drug use is increasing among females. Because steroids are male sex hormones, their effect in women is to make them more like men, including deeper voices, unwanted facial hair, breast shrinkage, and enlarged clitoris. However, many female athletes have discovered that even a small amount of testosterone can make a big difference in sports performance. That may let some female athletes remain competitive at an age when the performance of other similarly talented competitors has declined. Or some may be able to advance to the next level of competition, something they were unable to do on their own. As women's sports become more competitive and cash-driven, the temptation for females to augment their muscle power can be a very powerful motivator.

CHAPTER 1

WHO USES STEROIDS AND WHY?

Who uses steroids? From where does information about users come, and how do we know that information is true? A currently popular myth holds that steroids were a fad drug. Drug testing cleaned the problem up, so the story goes, and now the only users are marginal athletes trying to hang on, or kids who are experimenting. This scenario is indeed a myth. There has been almost no decrease in the amount of steroids and other illegal performance-enhancing drugs that are being used by athletes looking for strength and power.

Although there has been an alleged small decline in the ranks of Division I male college athletes who use steroids, the number of women athletes who use steroids has grown, a worrisome fact because they are the ones most vulnerable to permanent damage. Moreover, the ranks of steroid users include many individuals who don't compete in any sport. Firemen, policemen, and military personnel sometimes use steroids. Personal trainers and other individuals who work in health clubs and gyms often take steroids to help them achieve a "buffed" look, and they may recommend steroids to their clients. Models, dancers, and even certain movie stars (men and women) have used steroids to improve their appearance. Many teenagers who try steroids are looking for a better body image, not help in sports performance. And the list goes on.

The continuing interest in physical development makes it unlikely that steroids will fade away. Contemporary culture has elevated muscles to an art form, as evidenced by motion picture ads and magazine covers. An entire genre of popular action films features film heroes with sculpted physiques and bulging muscles that they use to great effect. Arnold Schwarzenegger, the prototype of the action hero, readily admits using steroids to achieve the look during his bodybuilding days, explaining that "everyone did it" back then. Today, the United States has more than 1 million current or former users of anabolic steroids. More than 300,000 of them used steroids within the past year. Almost none of them were under medical supervision, despite the known potential for negative short-term effects on physical and mental well-being.

Anabolic steroids do have uses as medical therapy, and they are prescribed for specific conditions. For example, they might be given to a weakened patient before or after surgery. Some hormonal problems can be corrected with steroids. They also have been tested successfully as a male contraceptive, and they are used routinely to fight the wasting associated with HIV and AIDS. There also seems to be a strong emerging trend toward using steroids as hormone replacement therapy in older men in much the same manner that estrogen is used for postmenopausal women. But this book is not directed at patients who receive steroids as legitimate medical therapy. The concern here is with those who are experimenting recklessly with their health and well-being and with those who are subverting the cause of sportsmanship by giving themselves an illegal edge in competition.

COUNTING THE USERS

How are steroid users counted? Until the late 1980s, very little data were available on who the users were. Most information was based on anecdotes, testimonials, and rumors. The true dimensions of the steroid problem in the United States were not known. The picture has changed since then, and important information has been gathered through several national surveys conducted by researchers at academic institutions and government agencies.

A 1988 study by William Buckley and Charles Yesalis was the first nationwide survey of anabolic steroid use among teenage boys. It showed that approximately 7 percent of high school seniors had used steroids. This study was prompted by anecdotal accounts from high school athletes, coaches, and athletic administrators that suggested that steroid use was much more widespread than had been previously documented, which proved to be the case. This research demonstrated that the wave of steroid use was spreading down (to younger kids) as well as out (to a greater number of kids). The results of that study have since been confirmed by more than 40 national, regional, and local studies.

William Anderson and Douglas McKeag, on behalf of the National Collegiate Athletic Association (NCAA), directed another landmark study that has provided much valuable information about steroid and other drug use by college student athletes. They surveyed more than 2,000 NCAA male and female athletes at 11 NCAA member colleges and universities about alcohol and drug use. This study, which began in 1985, has since been repeated twice.

The Youth Risk and Behavior Surveillance System (YRBSS) monitors health risk behaviors among youth—including use of alcohol, tobacco, and other drugs—through a national school-based survey of 9th through 12th graders. The YRBSS, which is sponsored by the Centers for Disease Control and Prevention (CDC), began in 1991 to collect information on anabolic steroid use. Since then, they have conducted a biennial survey of thousands of students—11,000 in the 1995 survey and 16,000 in the 1993 survey.

Monitoring the Future is another highly respected national survey of drug abuse conducted yearly on approximately 16,000 high school seniors. This study has measured steroid use since 1989.

The figure of 1 million U.S. steroid users comes from data collected by the National Household Survey on Drug Abuse (NHSDA), which provides information on individuals over the age of 12 in U.S. households. A sophisticated method of selecting a representative sample of the population is used, and this yearly survey is considered a gold standard for measuring drug use.

Persons participating in the survey are interviewed in their homes, and parents of respondents under age 18 may remain in the room during the interview. To promote anonymity, drug use questions are answered by marking a self-administered answer sheet. Substantially higher prevalence rates for use of some drugs (including anabolic steroids) in both the Monitoring the Future Study and the YRBSS have been attributed to youths being more willing to admit to use in the relative privacy of the school setting than they are at home where their parents may be present. Although only one survey

(NHSDA) specifically identifies the substance of interest as anabolic steroids (Monitoring the Future and YRBSS use the term steroids), all three surveys specify the nonmedical use of steroids that differentiates performance-enhancement steroids from those used for medicinal therapy.

The following sections examine how these five important studies were conducted and what they found.

Buckley/Yesalis Study

The study sample in the Buckley/Yesalis study was drawn from a pool of 150 schools across the nation that employed certified athletic trainers. Because only 12 percent of U.S. high schools had certified athletic trainers, the schools didn't represent a random sample of all U.S. high schools, but the sample schools did share the characteristics of a large number of U.S. schools. The schools were stratified into eight categories based on whether they were urban or rural, large or small, and Sunbelt or non-Sunbelt locales. (The latter category was used because anecdotal accounts put the rate of steroid use higher in the Sunbelt, which is defined as contiguous states that border the ocean or Mexico from Virginia south and west to Texas, Arizona, New Mexico, and California.) The questionnaires were administered to senior male students by their homeroom teachers and collected by the athletic trainer, who forwarded them to the researchers.

One finding of the study was that the user group tended to be chronologically older (but under age 19) than the non-user group, with greater minority representation in the user group. Respondents in the non-user group were more likely to have a parent who finished high school. Users were more likely to participate in school-sponsored athletics, specifically in football and wrestling. However, a revealing point of interest was that 35 percent of the user group did not intend to participate in any school-sponsored sport activities. Of the steroid users, approximately 58 percent judged their strength above average, whereas only 28 percent of non-users thought that. More steroid users (40 percent) reported their overall health to be excellent than did non-users (24 percent).

More than a third of the users (38 percent) said that their first steroid use occurred at age 15 or younger, and another third had started by age 16 (see figure 1.1). Users reported taking from one to more than five cycles of steroid use, with each cycle usually lasting

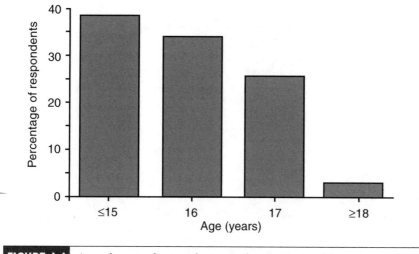

FIGURE 1.1 Age of respondents at first use of anabolic steroids.
Reprinted, by permission, from the American Medical Association, 1988.

6 to 12 weeks. Some 44 percent of users said they used more than one steroid at the same time (a practice known as stacking), and 38 percent had used both oral and injectable anabolic steroids.

Users were asked why they took steroids, and 47 percent said their main reason was to improve athletic performance (see figure 1.2). However, 27 percent said that appearance was their main reason. A particularly significant finding of this study is that approximately a quarter of teen steroid users report behaviors, perceptions, and opinions that are consistent with psychological dependence. These include an unwillingness to stop use, a misperception of the risks and benefits of use, and rationalization of drug use.

Anderson/McKeag Study

The 1985 Michigan State study by Anderson and McKeag showed that the heaviest steroid use (defined as having occurred within the past year) was among NCAA football players (9 percent). This figure does not seem unreasonable because many college players believe they are good enough to make the pros and view the economic promise of the NFL as a justification for their steroid use. Four percent of the male participants in track and field reported steroid use. Overall, 5 percent of Division I athletes, both male and female,

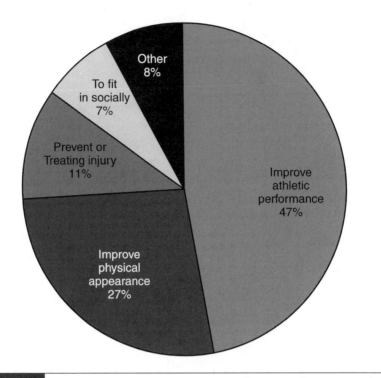

FIGURE 1.2   The most commonly cited reason for steroid use is improved athletic performance.

Adapted, by permission, from the American Medical Association, 1988.

4 percent of Division II athletes, and 2 percent of Division III athletes had used steroids within the 12 months prior to the study.

Anderson and McKeag repeated their study during the 1988-89 academic year and found steroid use had increased slightly over the intervening four years. Although steroid use remained at 5 percent for Division I athletes, the use among Division II athletes rose to 5 percent, and Division III use went to 4 percent. Again, the highest incidence of reported steroid use was among football players (10 percent). Steroid use remained at 4 percent for men's track and field events, but declined in baseball (2 percent) and in tennis (2 percent).

In 1993, the Michigan State study was repeated once more. This time, a significant decline in steroid use was observed among male athletes, although football players continued to have the highest level of self-reported use (5 percent). Female athletes, however, showed considerable increases in steroid use relative to the earlier two studies.

Youth Risk and Behavior Surveillance System

This study has shown that from 1991 to 1995, the proportion of adolescent males who reported past or present steroid use increased slightly from 4.1 percent to 4.9 percent, a change that is not statistically significant. Likewise, although the proportion of adolescent females who reported past or present use doubled from 1.2 percent in 1991 to 2.4 percent in 1995, the increase is not statistically significant.

Monitoring the Future Study

Although the 1991 Monitoring the Future survey disclosed an overall significant drop from 1989-1990 steroid use levels, steroid use has remained essentially steady among male seniors since then, with about 4 percent admitting to using steroids at some time in their life. Also noteworthy is the fact that female steroid use has increased significantly over the past several years, from approximately 0.5 percent to 1 percent. Other studies have confirmed this fact.

NHSDA Study

The data in the NHSDA study show that males have much higher levels of steroid use over a lifetime than females. Although the median age for first use is 18 years, many 12- to 17-year-olds have taken anabolic steroids. There have been well-founded reports of steroid use even among fifth graders. The NHSDA data also established that the use of steroids was significantly associated with the use of other illicit drugs, cigarettes, and alcohol. In particular, adolescent steroid users are three to four times more likely to use alcohol or cigarettes than non-users.

Further, steroid use was highly correlated with self-reported aggressive behavior and crimes against property. Eighty-three percent of adolescent users (versus 38 percent of non-users) admitted to having been involved in a physical confrontation during the previous year, including fighting, armed robbery, or using physical force to obtain something. Likewise, 80 percent of users (versus 27 percent of non-users) acknowledged committing a crime against property, such as robbery or vandalism.

Validity of the Studies

A point of concern frequently expressed is whether we can believe these studies. Were the answers truthful, particularly with regard to adolescent use? Perhaps some non-users claim to take steroids so they will appear to be more sophisticated or worldly. Is there a brag factor? Certainly, this issue is a matter of concern for all researchers who must design their studies to elicit honest answers as well as they can. For instance, the NHSDA, Monitoring the Future, and YRBSS questionnaires are self-administered and anonymous surveys, so there is little incentive to lie.

Underreporting is also an issue of concern. For instance, researchers were skeptical when 39 percent of the males and 56 percent of the females in a 1988 study of high school athletes denied ever hearing of using anabolic steroids to enhance sports performance. This lack of awareness appeared to be unusual considering that the study took place at a time when the media was giving great attention to the steroid problem.

The results of the nationwide study of high school steroid use by Buckley and Yesalis have been validated in part by other studies of various populations that used somewhat different methods to gather data but came up with similar findings. Other studies that confirmed the Buckley/Yesalis research found that between 4 percent and 12 percent of high school boys admit to using steroids at some time in their life. Some of the studies examined anabolic steroid use by high school girls and usually found that about .5 to 2 percent of high school girls report having used them. More recently, a study of seventh grade students in Modesto, California found that 5 percent of males and 3 percent of females admitted using steroids. As you will see in chapter 4, "Health Consequences of Steroid Use," these numbers are cause for concern.

In summary, most observers believe that some overreporting of steroid use may occur but that it is unlikely to be enough to bias test results. They agree that respondents more likely underreport steroid use so as to meet socially acceptable standards of behavior. Young athletes, especially collegiate athletes, are unlikely to be frank about using anabolic steroids when their use is a violation of the rules of virtually all the sports federations, as well as being against the traditional ethics of fair play in sports.

In fact, some experts question whether the recently reported decrease in steroid use among NCAA athletes is real or whether athletes are merely trying to protect the reputation of their sport. The continued increase in the size and strength of college football players flies in the face of any reported decline in steroid use. Some people contend that increasingly aggressive drug testing of collegiate athletes has led to a drop in steroid use, but the increase in the level of use among women would argue against that contention.

PORTRAIT OF A STEROID USER

The preponderance of research demonstrates that the pattern of drug use for various substances is most likely to develop between the ages of 11 and 24 years. Data from national, state, and local surveys clearly and consistently show that steroid use is present in grades 7 through 12. Thus, any effort to stop steroid use in sports must begin with younger children.

At a conference in Prague, an agent of the California State Bureau of Narcotic Enforcement stated that a typical profile has emerged for non-athlete adult users of anabolic steroids. The typical steroid user is a white male, 18-45 years old (but most likely in the range of 25-30), who may have a part-time, minimum-wage job, a high school education or less, and has only a minor criminal record. He likely uses many drugs, including tranquilizers, codeine products, marijuana, and associated non-steroid anabolic agents like chromium picolinate and creatinine. He differs markedly from the competitive athlete user, who typically takes steroids in cycles, by using steroids in an uninterrupted fashion. Also, he normally obtains his steroids from distributors in the black market rather than from legitimate medical sources.

You may wonder why steroid use by athletes hasn't dropped sharply since its health risks have been documented. The answer for some appears to be that the perceived benefits outweigh the risks. Other users are convinced that the news media has sensationalized the risks. Although there may be some truth to that assertion, these drugs are far from harmless. Because steroids have been shown to make some users more aggressive, there is concern about the mechanism of aggression. With young users, inappropriate aggressive behavior may be a direct result of taking steroids, or it may be part of a pattern of excessive risk-taking. Experts do agree, however, that adding an outside hormonal boost at a peak time of naturally occurring hormonal change is unwise at the very least.

Bodybuilders and Steroids

One group of steroid users about whom we have little information other than a few surveys and numerous anecdotal accounts are the bodybuilders and "gym rats" who comprise the physical training/drug-taking culture. Although bodybuilding involves hard work and is physically demanding, the contests where the results are displayed could almost be described as beauty contests. Moreover, the large majority of individuals who bodybuild seldom, if ever, compete.

The inherent problem with bodybuilding is that when development of the body becomes a person's main focus, it is easy to develop a narcissistic preoccupation with the physical self that can distort reality. This preoccupation happens in much the same way that other body image disorders, such as anorexia, distort body image. One Harvard researcher coined the term *reverse anorexia* to describe a condition wherein an individual believes he is not muscular when, in fact, any rational person would see him as very muscular.

Researchers know that the users in this group will have the most trouble discontinuing steroids because giving up steroids often means abandoning an entire lifestyle (see chapter 8). Studying this group of steroid users in a scientific manner has been difficult, but a handful of surveys suggest that the level of steroid use is very high and ranges from 20 percent to more than 50 percent in men and 3 percent to more than 10 percent in women. However, in professional or elite competitive bodybuilding, the level of steroid use (defined as use at some point in a lifetime) is believed to be at or near 100 percent.

WHY ATHLETES USE STEROIDS

At the time steroid use was spreading through the ranks of athletes in diverse sports during the 1960s and early '70s, little thought was given, at least by the athletes, to either the health risk or whether such drug use was ethical. Many athletes viewed steroids simply as a major training aid, similar to how vitamins and other dietary supplements are viewed today. In addition to looking for a competitive "edge," athletes feared that not using the drug would put them at a disadvantage. For example, at the elite level in sprinting, time differences of less than a half second may define whether an athlete is successful or an also-ran.

STEVE COURSON

Steve Courson is a former steroid user who has become an effective and outspoken critic of drug use in sport. As an offensive lineman for the Pittsburgh Steelers in their glory days of the 1970s and early 1980s, Courson was inside the NFL as steroid use swept through the sport. He recalls that his own steroid use began in college where the drugs were prescribed by a team physician and paid for by his university. "It was somewhat secretive behavior then," he says, "but people would tell you honestly if they used."

Courson was a man of legendary strength; he dominated the NFL Strongest Man competitions from 1980 to 1982 and once bench-pressed 605 pounds. He believes steroids gave him an edge in developing his strength and power. Since leaving the NFL, however, Courson has had a lot of time to think about the negative health effects of steroids, including heart disease, during his struggle to regain his formerly robust health and stay off the list for a heart transplant. Does he have regrets now about his steroid use? "I have regrets that I sold out to the system," he says frankly, "that I was so gung ho that I turned myself into a biochemical machine and complied with the 'win at all costs' directive."

Courson maintains that he took steroids so that he could compete on an even basis with the many other steroid users in professional football. He scoffs at the popular media portrayal of a pro football steroid user as someone who uses drugs to make up for lack of ability. "It was a reflection of your commitment to football," he explains. "You're hurt and they want you to play. Are you committed enough to use steroids? It's a sad thing because you can't be honest about that kind of commitment."

Like many other professional athletes, Courson stopped taking steroids when his football career ended. What he did not know was the damage his body had sustained. This thoughtful, literate former NFL Super Bowl competitor now coaches high school football players who can talk frankly to him about drugs and sports. He freely tells them that while using steroids was the right decision from a performance stand-point, it was wrong as an ethical decision and had serious health consequences.

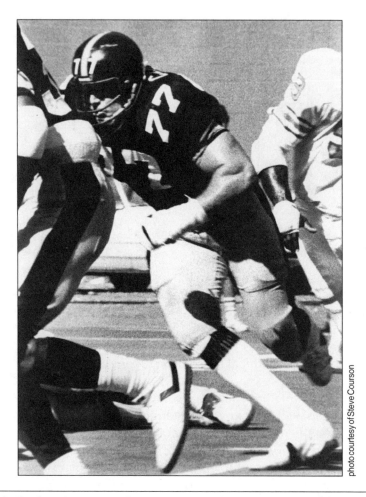

photo courtesy of Steve Courson

Now a high school football coach, Steve Courson (77), a former steroid user and NFL star, tells kids that using steroids is ethically wrong and has serious health consequences.

Consider the example of Ben Johnson, the Canadian sprinter who won the gold medal in the 100 meter sprint on a hot August afternoon at the 1988 Olympic Games in Seoul, South Korea, and then lost it because of a positive test for steroids. Although nobody can quantify how much steroids helped Johnson, he was the best ever while he was using them—his best time is still unequaled. After his suspension from competition was lifted, Johnson attempted a comeback but never again attained anything like his previous drug-aided times.

Some will argue that he was older and had been away from competition at the world level for too long when he made his comeback attempt, and there is no doubt those factors played a role, just as there is no doubt that steroids gave him an edge. Many believe that every athlete on the track with Johnson that day had, at one time or another, used banned drugs, and that Johnson was just unlucky in getting caught. The real story may never be known. An anonymous Soviet coach was quoted in The New York Times in October 1988 as saying, "I feel sorry for Ben Johnson. All sportsmen—not all, but maybe 90 percent, including our own—use drugs."

The question then is what becomes of the 10 percent the Soviet coach says aren't using drugs. Will they be able to win medals anyway, or will they be coerced into taking dangerous drugs to stay even? Because steroids fundamentally alter athletic competitions, Olympians who don't take steroids nevertheless have a keen interest in the subject. Greg Barton, a double Olympic gold medalist in kayaking, disapproves of steroid use. He has said he knew of several European paddlers who were using steroids and that this was a source of concern to him at almost every world-level meet. Would he be able to sustain his success while competing against people who used drugs? The pressure to use drugs may begin very early with gifted athletes. In 1995, a 14-year-old girl from South Africa had a positive steroid test and was banned from international competition in track and field for two years.

THE SPREAD OF STEROID USE

The Russian weight lifters of the 1950s are credited with being the first athletes to compete internationally on steroids. In 1954, Dr. John Ziegler, physician for the U.S. weight lifting team, reportedly was advised by his Soviet counterpart that the Russian weight lifters were taking testosterone. As soon as Ziegler returned to the U.S., he tried testosterone himself and then gave it to several New York weight lifters.

Anabolic steroid use probably was limited to the Soviet and American weight lifters at the 1960 Olympic Games, but after they sang the praises of the drugs, the throwers in track and field became converts. By the mid-1960s, most of the top-ranking throwers had tried steroids, including Randy Matson, the 1968 Olympic champion and world-record holder in the shot put; Dallas Long, the 1964 Olympic shot put champion; Harold Connolly, the 1956 Olympic champion in the hammer throw; and Russ Hodge, a world-record holder in the decathlon. By 1968, many sprinters, hurdlers, and middle-distance runners were taking steroids.

The morality or propriety of using steroids was not even an issue and the only discussion of them at the Games was about which ones worked best. Most users were fairly open about their activities. Bill Toomey, gold medalist in the decathlon at the 1968 Olympics and winner of the prestigious Sullivan Award given by the Amateur Athletic Union, freely admitted his performance was drug-aided. A survey of track and field athletes (including U.S. athletes) participating in the 1972 Olympic Games revealed that 68 percent reported prior steroid use and 61 percent had used steroids within the past six months.

In 1971, after he won a gold medal at the Pan American Games in Cali, Colombia, weight lifter Ken Patera talked about his upcoming meeting with Russian superheavyweight Vasily Alexeev in the 1972 Olympics in Munich in an interview in the Los Angeles Times. "Last year," Patera said, "the only difference between me and him was I couldn't afford his drug bill. Now I can. When I hit Munich I'll weigh in at about 340 or maybe 350. Then we'll see which are better, his steroids or mine."

When steroid use spread to female athletes, sports events of the mid-1960s took on an odd cast as many individuals who came to the starting blocks of female events appeared very masculine in their shape, stance, and voice. There was speculation that Eastern Bloc countries had resorted to using men disguised as women or hermaphrodites (individuals with characteristics of both sexes). The ensuing uproar led to the initiation of sex testing in 1967 at the European Cup. Several female athletes did fail the screening, and a few others retired from competition. It seems clear now that the large majority of these masculinized women had been given some form of anabolic steroids. The spread of steroids among female athletes followed the male pattern, beginning with the strength athletes and then to others in track and field. Steroid use has since diffused into other sports, having been reported at the collegiate level in basketball, swimming, gymnastics, lacrosse, and softball.

Professional football players embraced steroids early on. In 1963, the San Diego Chargers hired Alvin Roy, a Baton Rouge gym owner who had been an assistant coach for the U.S. weight lifting team, to be their strength coach. Some former Chargers later said they were not told what the "little pink pills" placed beside their plates at the

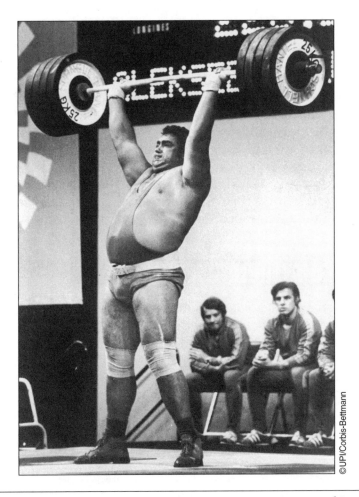

©UPI/Corbis-Bettmann

(Vasily Alexeev) In an attempt to compete and win at elite levels, some athletes and teams may use steroids to boost their performance.

training table were, but that there was a clear implication they would be fined for refusing to take them. Steroid use spread quickly from team to team. Pat Donovan, a Dallas Cowboy offensive lineman who retired in 1983, said "Anabolic steroids are very, very accepted in the NFL. In my last five or six years, it (steroid use) ran as high as 60 percent to 70 percent on the Cowboys on the offensive and defensive lines."

There was no early official reaction as steroids spread through sports. Doctors played a role in "selling" the drugs by first praising them and then by prescribing them. Until the late 1980s, doctors were the primary source of the drugs for more than a third of the users in the United States. Today, less than 10 percent of steroid users obtain their drugs by prescription.

Doctors, to their credit, also were among the first to realize that steroids were not just a fountain of youth drug but had the potential for harm. However, a schism that developed between doctors and athletes (see chapter 3) meant that the former often were not the first line of information about steroids. Athletes began experimenting with combinations of steroids taken together and in sequence, a practice known as stacking. There also was simultaneous use of oral and injected steroids. Potential users looked to muscle magazines, underground publications, and current or former users. Articles in

FINDING STEROID USERS

Because anabolic steroids are primarily training drugs, drug testing that occurs at announced intervals is highly ineffective in detecting users. For instance, the NCAA began testing for anabolic steroids at football bowl games and championship events in 1986. Results from this announced drug testing showed that between 1 and 2 percent of athletes used anabolic steroids, a fairly low percentage. These results led the public to conclude that steroid use was confined to a very small group of elite athletes.

In 1984 and 1985, the United States Olympic Committee (USOC) conducted a series of unannounced drug tests at a number of Olympic sports events. Approximately 50 percent of athletes tested positive! No sanctions (punishments) were imposed for positive results in this series of tests, which was intended to gather information about athlete drug use.

An obvious conclusion that can be drawn is that the results of previously scheduled drug tests at athletic events are a poor indicator of the overall incidence of anabolic steroid use. Moreover, the effectiveness of out-of-competition testing was brought into question by the successes of the East German and Chinese athletes. What is apparent is that many athlete steroid users have access to sophisticated information on dosage regimens and washout times. The usage levels discovered at these nonpunitive unannounced tests lead to the conclusion that athletes remain convinced that taking anabolic steroids will enhance their sports performance.

the media about steroid use among athletes were a mixed blessing. Although they brought the problem to public attention, they also served to drive it underground.

The reaction of sports organizations was slow in coming and took different forms. In the Eastern Bloc countries of Europe, the governments and sports federations institutionalized steroid use. U.S. sports federations always have had a public anti-drug stance, although they have sometimes been accused of helping user athletes by blocking effective drug testing programs or covering up positive test results. The first full-scale drug testing for anabolic steroids took place at the 1976 Summer Games in Montreal. More than 10 years would pass before the NCAA instituted drug testing. Early drug tests did not look at testosterone esters (an injectable form of testosterone which, after entering the blood, is indistinguishable from natural testosterone) until 1982 because the testing technology was not available.

Professional sports organizations have struggled with the problem over the past 20 years. Many say that they were caught unaware by the speed with which the steroid problem developed, but other observers attribute their actions to darker motives. Most federations first denied the existence of a problem, sometimes even when their own athletes were giving embarrassing public testimonials to the contrary. Next came in-competition testing, even though the limitations were already known. This testing was followed by pronouncements that the problems had been handled. When it became apparent that the problem hadn't been handled, sports federations switched to a random, year-round, out-of-competition program. It could be considered a triumph of hope over experience for the federations to pin their hopes on this program since it was already known that the new drug testing method contained numerous loopholes.

COMMENTS BY DR. Y

Steroid use among adolescents is not limited to the United States. Other countries, including Canada, England, Sweden and South Africa, have reported steroid use among their young people at levels similar to the United States. Drug testing conducted by laboratories approved by the International Olympic Committee (IOC) has documented steroid use among athletes from many of the 170 or so countries that participate in the Olympic movement. Although focusing on the multicultural aspect of the Olympic Games is fashionable, I believe that people are more alike than different, and some of these similarities account for the fact that steroid use is observed throughout the world.

Almost all cultures place high value on strength and muscularity among males. This value might take the form of adulation, a position of leadership, financial rewards, or a more attractive mate. Likewise, most cultures exhibit some competitive tendencies, as demonstrated by the rapid growth of the number of countries participating in the Olympic movement during the past 50 years. Most cultures also value winners more than losers. These attitudes have always posed a stumbling block to prevention efforts in that the positive effects of anabolic steroids are consistent with some of our basic cultural values.

CHAPTER 2

ALL ABOUT STEROIDS

An important first step in combating steroid use is understanding exactly what steroids are and how they were developed, how they work, and how athletes use them. Anabolic steroids are not mysterious wonder drugs; they are simply man-made versions of the primary male sex hormone, testosterone.

Hormones are one of the body's major regulatory mechanisms. Both men and women have natural hormones that serve as the controllers of the almost infinite number of chemical reactions that take place within our bodies. Hormones actively "turn on" or "turn off" a gene so as to alter the supply of cell components or influence the rate of chemical processes in the body. For example, hormones can tell muscle cells to produce specific proteins from raw materials within the body so that muscle tissue mass will increase. Hormones also can activate genes in skin cells to influence the growth of facial hair. Hormones regulate the supply of raw materials within the cells and often work directly to speed up or slow down certain biochemical reaction rates.

Two organs in the brain, the pituitary and the hypothalamus, control many hormonal functions. The thyroid gland and the pancreas also produce hormones. The group of hormones that are produced by the adrenal gland and ovaries in women, and the adrenal gland and testes in men, consist of a special type of lipid (fat) called steroids, which comes from a Greek word that means solid. The human body is capable of producing more than 600 different types of steroids, including testosterone, and a number of them exhibit male hormone-like activities. This family of compounds is known as androgens. The word androgen is derived from the Greek roots andro (meaning male) and gen (meaning to produce) and refers to male sex hormones.

The natural supply of testosterone in adult males is produced by the Leydig cells located within the testes. (Women and young boys do have a small amount of testosterone in their bodies that is produced by the adrenal gland.) Very little testosterone is stored within the body so that production must be more or less continuous. Testosterone is responsible for both the androgenic (masculinizing) and anabolic (tissue-building) effects that take place during puberty and continue in adulthood. It is the significant increase in the production of testosterone in a young male that precipitates puberty.

When testosterone exerts its effects in a pubescent male, the androgenic effect is responsible for an increase in the length and diameter of the penis, increased sex drive, and the appearance of pubic, axillary, and facial hair. The anabolic effects of testosterone during puberty include an increase in height, deepening of the voice, and an increase in muscle mass and strength, along with a decrease in body fat. All these changes take place without any physical exercise or training.

The principal reason for the difference in outward appearance of males and females (other than genitals and pelvic shape) is that males produce approximately 10 to 15 times more testosterone than women. Thus, testosterone is the primary substance that makes men look like men, and the absence of high levels of testosterone makes women look like women. This point is well-illustrated by looking at many of today's women bodybuilders who have altered their body shape by taking steroids, causing it to become masculine in appearance.

Anabolic steroids are primarily a consequence of research to develop drugs that would separate the tissue-building capability of testosterone from its masculinizing properties. This separation has never been fully achieved. Consequently, the proper name for this class of hormones is anabolic-androgenic steroids, although they are usually referred to simply as anabolic steroids or steroids.

Don't confuse anabolic steroids with corticosteroids such as prednisone or cortisone. Corticosteriods are hormones produced by the adrenal glands, and their biological properties are quite different from those of anabolic steroids. Corticosteroids like prednisone or cortisone are potent anti-inflammatory drugs used in medicine to treat conditions such as asthma and muscle strains and sprains. Their effect is catabolism (protein metabolism or breakdown) rather than anabolism (tissue protein building).

HOW ATHLETES TAKE STEROIDS

Anabolic steroids can be taken either by mouth, by injection, or, more recently, by skin creams or patches. If an individual simply swallowed a dose of testosterone, however, it would be quickly inactivated by the process of metabolism and cleared from the body through the liver. Steroids that are taken orally have had their chemical structure altered to slow their removal from the body by the liver but are more toxic to the liver. Steroids taken by intramuscular injection or skin application also have been chemically altered to slow their release into circulation.

Anabolic steroids have traditionally been taken in cycles, which are episodes of use lasting 6 to 12 weeks or more. Athletes often take more than one steroid at a time in a fashion known as stacking. In an attempt to avoid developing a tolerance to a particular anabolic steroid (plateauing), some users stagger their drugs, taking different anabolic steroids in an overlapping pattern, or they will stop taking one drug and start another. Steroid users often will pyramid their administration patterns, moving from a low daily dose at the beginning of the cycle to a higher dose, and then tapering the dose back down toward the end of the cycle. It should be noted that none of these steroid administration strategies has been shown to be effective.

In addition, individuals may use other drugs concurrently with anabolic steroids to counteract some of the common adverse effects of steroids. These drugs include diuretics (to handle fluid retention), antiestrogens (to prevent "breast" development, called gynecomastia), human chorionic gonadotrophin (to prevent testicular atrophy), and anti-acne medications. This type of polypharmacy is called an array. The frequency of this multiple drug use and the frequency of the steroid administration patterns described above are poorly documented.

The dosage of anabolic steroids taken depends on the sport as well

DIET AND STEROID USE

Many researchers have been keenly interested in the association of steroids and other drugs with dietary supplements and special diets. Most steroid users are on special diets, usually ones containing high levels of protein. In addition, steroid users frequently take dietary supplements such as vitamins, amino acids, minerals, garlic, protein powders, and creatine. Some use "steroid replacers" (substances taken during the user's off-steroids portion of the cycle) including chromium picolinate, glandular extracts, vanadyl sulfate, boron, DHEA, and smilax. (The worth of these dietary supplements and "steroid replacers" as performance enhancers has not been scientifically established, with the exception of creatine and DHEA). Anabolic steroid users commonly take other performance-enhancing drugs such as human growth hormone, human chorionic gonadotropin (hCG), clenbuterol, and amphetamines as well. Oftentimes, steroid users also use mood-altering drugs including alcohol, marijuana, cocaine, and tobacco.

as on the perceived needs of the athlete. Male endurance athletes use steroids primarily for their alleged effect of lowering recuperation time between workouts, and they use dosages at or slightly below what the body normally produces, about 7 milligrams a day of testosterone. Although sprinters desire similar results, the strength and power requirements of their activity result in dosages that are approximately 1.5 to 2 times normal levels.

Participants in the traditional strength sports who are seeking to "bulk up" have generally used dosages that exceed the body's normal production by 10 to 100 times or more. Administration patterns vary among athletes within a particular sport, based on each athlete's training goals, how he responds to the drugs, and on the presumed physiologic effects of different anabolic steroids. Women, regardless of sport, are generally thought to use lower dosages of anabolic steroids than men because it takes less for them to obtain the desired effect.

MECHANISMS OF ACTION

As was stated earlier, anabolic steroids were adopted initially by athletes in power sports such as weight lifting and football to increase strength and muscularity. From the beginning, these athletes consistently reported that the drugs also reduced their recovery time between workouts. That meant that they were able to work out more frequently, for longer periods of time, and with greater intensity. These observations by athletes very likely played an important role in the diffusion of anabolic steroids among sprinters in a variety of sports and, thereafter, to endurance athletes.

The truth is that anabolic steroids work. That is to say that anabolic steroids, especially when used in conjunction with intense strength training, increase muscle mass and strength well beyond what can be achieved with training alone. (Chapter 3 details these results.) Experts have suggested the following mechanisms to explain the performance-enhancing effects of anabolic steroids (see figure 2.1):

- An increase in protein synthesis
- Prevention of muscle tissue destruction caused by heavy work or exercise
- The effects on the central nervous system and the neuromuscular junctions
- Increased aggressiveness
- The placebo effect

How anabolic steroids work is most likely explained by a combination of these mechanisms.

Protein Synthesis and Cellular Repair

In the normal way of things, two things can happen when athletes such as wrestlers, runners, or swimmers stress their bodies through training at high levels of intensity over prolonged periods. First, their natural production of testosterone can drop precipitously, often to levels as low as those of a castrated man. Second, the body responds by releasing another type of steroid called glucocorticoids, which are not anabolic (tissue building) but catabolic, meaning that they break down muscle tissue. A popular theory holds that a visible sign of overtraining is muscle wasting.

Although the evidence is incomplete, scientists have speculated that anabolic steroids inhibit or block the catabolic effects of these glucocorticoids. If this theory is correct, a runner could endure more miles of road work per week and consequently lower her times, or a

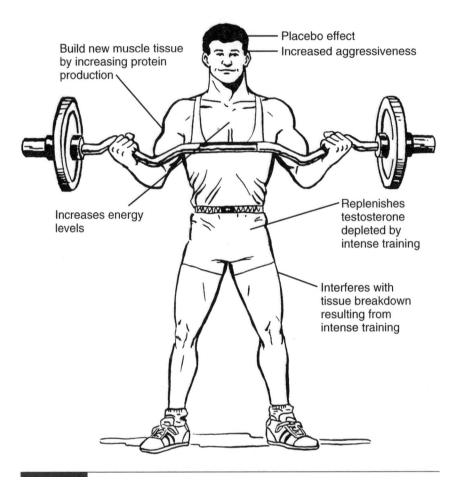

Build new muscle tissue
by increasing protein
production

Placebo effect
Increased aggressiveness

Increases energy
levels

Replenishes
testosterone
depleted by
intense training

Interferes with
tissue breakdown
resulting from
intense training

FIGURE 2.1   Steroid use allows a user to build more muscle tissue and become
stronger, but steroid use can have harmful consequences to the body
as well.

weight lifter could work out more often and do more sets and reps
and achieve greater muscle and strength gains. Some experts have
gone so far as to theorize that this anticatabolic mechanism may be
the most important factor in untangling the performance effects of
anabolic steroids. Beyond helping negate the muscle breakdown
effects of glucocorticoids, anabolic steroids help replenish testosterone levels depleted by intense training.

The anabolic effect of steroids comes through increasing protein
synthesis through their attachment to receptors in target tissues,
which include skeletal and heart muscle, skin, testes, prostate, and
various areas of the brain. Then these newly formed hormone

receptor complexes interact with other receptor sites on the chromo-
somes and, through this hormonal chain action, ultimately result in
the formation of various enzyme, structural (bone), and contractile
(muscle) proteins (see figure 2.2). Obviously, the effect on muscle
growth is of the greatest interest to steroid users. An "overload" of
anabolic steroids causes an increase in the production of proteins,
which in turn become building blocks for new cells.

The response to anabolic steroids, both positive and negative,
varies significantly among men and women. With regard to skeletal
muscle, anabolic steroids have a significantly greater impact on
females (young and old), old males, and prepubescent males than
they do on young adult males. Even within these groups there is
variation in muscle response to anabolic steroids, most likely due to
variations among individuals in the proportion of slow-twitch and
fast-twitch muscle fibers (individuals with a higher percentage of
fast-twitch fibers demonstrate greater response). Furthermore, even

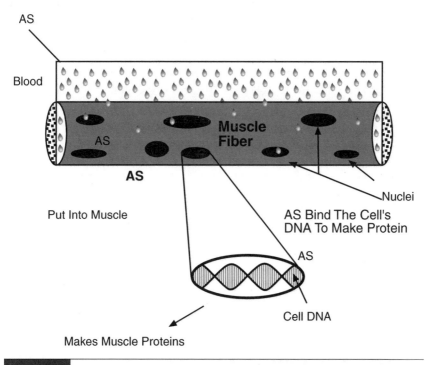

FIGURE 2.2   Oral and injectable anabolic steroids get to the muscle via the blood
and interact with the genetic machinery (DNA) to make more
contractile proteins (muscle).

Data courtesy of Dr. William Kraemer.

though all skeletal muscles respond to anabolic steroids, the sensitivity of individual muscles to steroids varies significantly. The pectoral muscles and shoulder girdle appear to be the most sensitive in males, probably because of the higher proportion of fast-twitch fibers in these muscle groups.

The Nervous System and Psychological Effects

Many steroid users have reported increased energy levels and aggressiveness. Researchers have used several different types of psychological testing to discover whether this change is a factor that could account for some performance gains that are attributed to steroids. Whereas much of the discussion of steroid-induced aggression has focused on the negative side, little attention has been paid to the fact that appropriately channeled increased aggression is a part of most of athletics. In fact, such aggression is valued in sports such as football and wrestling because, in the eyes of many coaches, it is associated with improved performance. Likewise, it is logical to assume that an athlete doing strength training or conditioning in a more aggressive manner and with more energy would achieve better results. In addition, there is a widely held belief that increased aggression allows an athlete to better tolerate the pain and discomfort associated with intense training.

Although studies have demonstrated that anabolic steroids can affect both the central nervous system and neuromuscular junctions, the relationship between these findings and the increased aggressiveness and energy levels reported by athletes is not well understood. These findings do, however, raise the possibility that there could be a biochemical foundation for the aggressiveness some steroid users display. A corollary to this theory is the assertion that when a large, heavily muscled individual acts in an aggressive manner, he will receive more attention than a small person who behaves aggressively, because the large man can do more damage.

The Placebo Effect

The term *placebo effect* refers to changes, either physical or psychological, that occur when an individual takes an inert substance that he believes will have a therapeutic effect. This medical phenomenon has been observed since the days of the ancient Greeks. Many people mistakenly believe that any benefit attributed to a placebo resides only in a person's imagination. This belief may hold true for some cases, but others have improvement based on objective clinical standards.

Although our understanding of the mind's effect on the body is still in its infancy, the effect is no less real. Thus, it seems likely that at least some athletes who take steroids see and realize gains because they expect to see them. Regardless of the mechanism, the overpowering response reported by athletes who use steroids over the past 40 years is far greater than what could be expected from the placebo effect alone, however.

How anabolic steroids actually work is most likely explained by a combination of the mechanisms that have been described here.

WHAT STEROIDS ARE NOT

Steroids are not instant muscles. If a young man takes steroids but does not maintain an adequate diet and fails to do rigorous strength training during the drug-taking cycle, he is unlikely to experience as many of the desired gains in muscle mass or strength. Even with intense training and a proper diet, the effects of steroids on males are much more variable and dependent on other circumstances. Steroids are not a substitute for athletic talent either. "You can't make chicken salad out of chicken feathers," goes the old saw. Things like timing, control, balance, and the ability to think clearly when events are happening quickly don't come from a bottle or an injection.

HOW STEROIDS WERE DEVELOPED

The search for the source of human strength is ancient. For hundreds of years before the word hormone came into the language, strength and power were linked with male sex organs. Primitive people commonly ate animal organs, sometimes even those of humans, in the belief that they could improve their strength, courage, or sexual function. As early as 140 BC, a healer in India advocated eating testicle tissue as a cure for impotence.

The practice of human castration, which probably originated

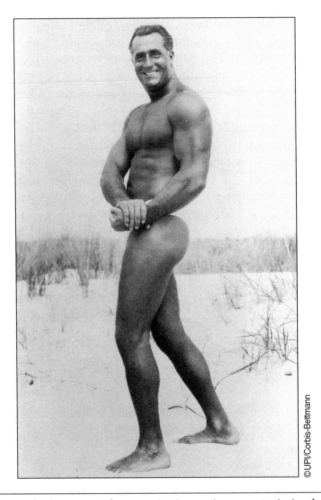

©UPI/Corbis-Bettmann

Charles Atlas in the 1940s and other popular figures for centuries before have made
a muscular body the ideal.

about 2000 BC in Babylon, provided evidence that loss of the testicles
meant that males lost not only their fertility, but also their strength,
their power, and their aggressiveness. Animal castration provided
similar evidence. Even though Aristotle (300 BC) knew nothing
about the secretion of sex hormones, he still was able to clearly
describe the effect of castration on a bird.

In 1889, a French physician named Charles-Edouard Brown-
Séquard performed a series of experiments in which he injected
extracts made from animal testes into dogs and even himself. He
reported an improvement in general health, muscular strength,

appetite, regulation of the intestinal tract, and mental faculties. This experiment was not scientifically controlled, and today his results have been attributed to the placebo effect. However, his work stimulated other researchers to follow in his footsteps. In the continuing quest for youth and vigor, injections of animal testicle extracts and even the surgical implantation of monkey testicles became very popular in mainstream medicine until the early 1930s. Thereafter, the practice dwindled and died out as a result of the work of responsible scientists who debunked these claims of rejuvenation.

Most scientists of the late 1700s and early 1800s believed that the nervous system was the mediator of the changes that occurred after castration. Then in 1849, a German scientist named Berthold did a simple but elegant experiment with six roosters. He showed that the changes in the combs and wattles that occurred when roosters were castrated could be prevented if the removed testes were transplanted into the bird's abdominal cavity. This experiment made it clear that the active masculinizing substance was produced in the bloodstream and did not involve the central nervous system.

Understanding Hormones

A burst of research activity that began in the 1920s on hormones and the endocrine system, and on male hormones specifically, led to an important series of observations about how hormonal control occurs, what it does, and which hormones are responsible for specific functions. By 1935, testosterone had been isolated, its chemical structure identified, and the basic nature of its anabolic and androgenic effects had been recognized.

The next major figure in hormonal research was the man most experts consider the father of anabolic steroids, Dr. Charles Kochakian. In the early 1930s, Dr. Kochakian showed that a hormone-like extract from male urine stimulated a strong positive nitrogen balance in castrated dogs. This finding was important because positive nitrogen balance indicates the synthesis of new tissue (proteins) in dogs and in humans. Thus, the anabolic or tissue-building properties of testosterone were established! A subsequent series of studies in rats showed similar results, and again, the positive nitrogen balance was associated with an increase in nonfat body weight.

Once researchers discovered that testosterone stimulates the protein-synthesizing or tissue-building process, it was immediately clear that there could be important medical applications if the tissue-building properties could be isolated. Throughout the 1940s, scientists grappled with the problem of getting the tissue-building effects of testosterone without also getting the masculinizing effects. The notion of a drug that could stimulate the development of new tissue was extremely attractive during World War II because it could aid in wound healing and perhaps save lives. Thus, the project took on new significance.

Dr. Kochakian soon became concerned about possible misuse of anabolic steroids, and he has warned that a complete split of the hormonal properties is not possible. "There is no such thing as a pure anabolic steroid," he has written. "All of the modified steroids still retain sufficient virilizing (masculinizing) activity to make them objectionable as therapeutic agents, especially in children and women."

While experiments to find a testosterone preparation that would stimulate tissue-building continued, other researchers worked to alter the chemical structure of testosterone. The addition of esters, which are formed from an alcohol and an acid when water is removed, was one method used to chemically alter the testosterone molecule. Some of these testosterone esters proved to be useful for treating protein deficiency in both humans and in horses. Almost 60 years later, these same testosterone esters are one of the chief drugs that athletes use.

From Laboratory to Reality

During the early 1940s, several researchers and a popular science writer of the day named Paul de Kruif observed that a drug that promoted tissue building would be very useful to athletes. In "The Male Hormone," de Kruif raised hopes and expectations for the newly synthesized anabolic steroids. He argued that these hormones had the potential to rejuvenate individuals and improve their productivity. With regard to athletes, de Kruif commented, "We know how both the St. Louis Cardinals and the St. Louis Browns have won championships supercharged by vitamins. It would be interesting to watch the productive power of an industry or a professional group (of athletes) that would try a systematic supercharge with testosterone."

De Kruif's popular scientific writings were not without effect.

TESTING THE DRUGS

One of the first tasks when a promising new drug is being developed is to track side effects, or unwanted results. The usual way to gather this type of information is for the manufacturer of a promising drug to test it for safety and efficacy, first in animals and then, if all goes well, in humans. During the clinical trials phase, the drug(s) is given to people who have been informed about potential side effects and risks and who have consented in writing. Careful records are maintained. A drug that has too many side effects may never get past the clinical trial stage.

Most of the legitimate medical uses of anabolic steroids have been established through clinical experiments, such as the use of anabolic steroids as a replacement therapy for men whose testes do not produce a normal amount of testosterone or their use as a male contraceptive agent. The results of these trials are available in the medical literature, that is, peer-reviewed medical journals. Now that researchers have gained more experience with anabolic steroids, it appears that the health risks parallel, in part, those associated with the use of female sex hormones for contraception. Birth control pills are a combination of estrogen and androgen that make conception unlikely if taken as directed. The health risks of birth control pills have been shown to be less than the health risks associated with pregnancy and therefore are considered an acceptable trade-off.

No presumed physical health benefit exists when a healthy young man elects to take steroids or other performance-enhancing drugs, however. Moreover, athletes often take far higher doses of anabolic steroids than have ever been given in clinical trials or for therapeutic reasons. In effect, they are running their own experiments with no scientific control. One problem with this type of freelance human study is that positive results are publicized among user groups, but serious side effects may be suppressed or, for that matter, exaggerated.

Another source of information about health effects from a drug are case reports in medical journals. Although by their very nature case reports can never establish a cause and effect relationship, they can be used to lay the foundation for more sophisticated epidemiologic research. If a physician knows that his patient is taking (or has taken) anabolic steroids and he believes the medical condition for which he is treating the patient is associated with that drug use, he may write a case report and submit it to a medical journal for publication. However, not all such episodes are formally chronicled by the attending physician and not all case reports get published. Those that do often deal with serious illness or death and usually involve an individual who is taking many times the therapeutic dosage of the drug.

Because many steroid users conceal their drug use from their doctors, some associations between drug use and adverse effects are never reported. Still another complicating and confounding issue is the fact that people who use anabolic steroids often take other drugs such as diuretics, thyroid hormone, growth hormone, cocaine, marijuana, tobacco, alcohol, and amphetamines. They may take megadoses of nutritional supplements or have a bizarre dietary regimen. What effect these combinations of other drugs and supplements have is unknown, and their interactions with steroids have never been studied scientifically.

Combined with the significant positive observations reported from clinical studies in professional journals, it was a relatively easy extrapolation for some in bodybuilding to assume that additional anabolic hormones would allow development of greater than normal body size. Still, no one knows exactly how steroids moved from the scientific realm into the world of sports. Some say that bodybuilders in California were using testosterone preparations as early as the latter 1940s; others say it was the Russian weight lifters of the early 1950s. What we do know is that even while researchers were still sorting out the mechanisms of action and testing drugs in a methodical fashion, steroid use jumped from the laboratory and began spreading through sports.

The truth is that we still don't know exactly how steroids do what they do in terms of athletic performance. Researchers who were using a variety of rodents, dogs, cats, monkeys, and domestic farm animals to study the effects of anabolic steroids found this testing was not helpful, even though the results were very consistent. Normal male animals who are exercised have consistently shown no increase in body weight or improvement in performance after treatment with anabolic steroids, but there is no way to perform sports testing with animals.

When scientists tried to establish the performance effects of anabolic steroids in human subjects, the results were contradictory and confusing. The problem was eventually traced to different research methods, but this early research on performance effects caused a great deal of misunderstanding between athletes and physicians. A number of doctors independently concluded that steroids were just a fad and so advised their patients. A minority of physicians and scientists realized early on the powerful effect that these drugs could have on human capabilities. Sadly, some medical professionals, both in this country and abroad, have played a significant role over the past 40 years in assisting athletes in the use of these drugs.

In a formal position statement in 1977, the American College of Sports Medicine (ACSM) concluded that anabolic steroids did not work. It explained that any weight gain was due to fluid retention associated with the drugs, and that any strength gain was the result of the placebo effect. This statement ran contrary to the overwhelming testimonials by athletes. By 1984, scientific data were available to cause the organization to reverse its position. The ACSM's earlier stance, however, caused it to lose credibility with athletes, a consequence that the organization still endures to some extent.

In retrospect, the athletes were convinced thoroughly of the beneficial effects of anabolic steroids several decades before there was consensus in the medical community that steroid use does result in strength and muscle gains beyond what would be expected from training alone. Chapter 3 discusses in detail how these conclusions were reached.

COMMENTS BY DR. Y

When you review the history of anabolic steroid use in sport and exercise, a number of ironies emerge. Not only did the medical community develop these drugs, but it played an early role in "selling" this potential fountain of youth. It was a physician, as well as some officials and supporters of the U.S. weight-lifting team, who initiated use of these drugs in this country. It was physicians who, until at least the late 1980s, served as the primary source of these drugs for more than one-third of the steroid users in this country. Often, it was physicians and/or coaching staffs at the professional, collegiate, or high school levels who provided, facilitated, or encouraged steroid use. Today, some physicians are in the vanguard of those who want to treat symptoms of male aging with testosterone.

Government scientists and sport federation officials institutionalized steroid use in Eastern Bloc countries and may have done the same thing in Communist China. In this country, the problem of steroid use fell to sport federations, which for decades covered it up, conveniently looked the other way, or instituted drug-testing programs that were designed to fail. As always, our society is the one that most emphasizes and rewards speed, strength, size, aggression, and winning.

CHAPTER 3

STEROID EFFECTS ON PERFORMANCE AND APPEARANCE

There is no doubt that anabolic steroids can have a major effect on both sports performance and appearance, but these effects cannot be exactly quantified. Taking steroids is not a cookbook procedure; different circumstances produce different results. The user's physiologic response to the drugs, the types of drugs taken, the combination, the sequence in which the drugs were taken, the length of use, the expectations of the user, and many other factors play a role in determining the drug's effects.

Females and young boys who use steroids do have certain predictable changes that may be permanent and not altogether pleasing. Nevertheless, the number of female steroid users is growing, especially among adolescents. The gains in strength that women get from steroids are so dramatic that it is often easier to see the performance-enhancing effects in women's competition rather than in men's, where the differences may be just enough to make the difference between receiving an Olympic medal and finishing in the pack.

In any event, sports performance itself is unpredictable. Outstanding athletic achievement occurs when many separate factors blend, and manipulating only one factor will almost never be enough to determine success. The ingredients for optimal athletic performance include genetic heritage, level of conditioning, skill, mental state or mind set, and diet. No amount of any drug can make up for poor conditioning or lack of skill.

If an athlete has all the necessary prerequisites for success, however, then manipulating one factor can be significant. Consider the stunning successes Chinese women athletes posted in swimming and in track and field several years ago before some of them were identified as users of anabolic steroids through positive drug tests. Their unlikely successes on the playing field had already raised the index of suspicion before these positive tests.

In an August 1993 article in *The Chicago Tribune*, Olympic reporter/ writer Phil Hersh described the end of the women's 10,000 meter race at the world track and field championships in Stuttgart, Germany. "After they crossed the finish line...the third, fourth, and fifth finishers lay on the track in pained exhaustion. At the same time, the first and second finishers, Wang Junzia, 20, and Zhong Huandi, 26, were taking a brisk victory lap with the Chinese flag." Hersh wrote that the ease with which the Chinese women ran the victory lap first stunned and then so irritated the crowd that it began to jeer the gold and silver medalists.

In November 1993, Hersh wrote about Chinese female swimmers, saying, "This year, the Chinese have made an unfathomable great leap forward, swamping the world rankings and reviving the East German (doping) nightmare for most of the swimming world. It is considered no coincidence that former East German coaches played a major role in building the foundation of women's swimming in China."

WHAT ATHLETES WANT FROM STEROIDS

Athletes want the following things from steroids:

- Alteration of body composition (increased muscle mass and reduced fat)
- Increased strength
- Increased endurance
- Faster recovery from exercise (so the athlete can perform longer, more frequent, or higher-intensity workouts)
- Enhanced athletic performance

PERFORMANCE EFFECTS

The quick answer to the question about whether steroids "work" is yes, but that is just a short answer to a complex question. Even though most of the athletic community accepts that steroids do enhance exercise capacity and performance, the extent to which these effects occur and the factors influencing such effects still is not clearly understood.

The two potential sources of information about steroid effects on performance and appearance are the scientific literature and the testimonials of users. The scientific literature includes studies of humans and animals that were performed according to generally accepted methods of scientific investigation. The problem is that results of these studies are inconsistent.

On the other hand, the testimonials from steroid users are highly consistent, but all anecdotal reports are somewhat questionable. (An anecdotal report is one person's account of what he thinks happened and thus is subject to sources of bias, such as the placebo effect.) Generally, researchers do not like to consider testimonials as data, even though they may provide interesting scientific leads. Nevertheless, even though such reports do not replace a base of accurate information gained from well-designed scientific studies, the large amounts of information obtained from the personal experiences of steroid users should not and cannot be ignored. Steroid users give themselves amounts and combinations of drugs that no ethical scientific investigator could ever do, especially not to women and adolescents.

Nor are animal studies particularly useful. Young male animals given steroids did not demonstrate any increase in body weight or improvement in performance after treatment. The problem may lie in trying to apply sports animal studies to humans. First, the types of exercise are not comparable (running on a treadmill or swimming for the animals versus strength training for humans). Second, there is no way to know whether the psychological effects of the human competitive drive can be simulated in animals. Therefore, the most relevant information about the effects of steroids comes from the human studies that have been conducted. These effects can be divided into three types: aerobic capacity and endurance, body composition, and strength performance.

Aerobic Capacity and Endurance

The theory is that because anabolic steroids stimulate bone marrow to produce more of the red blood cells that carry oxygen, an athlete could expect to get an increase in aerobic endurance performance. The maximal oxygen uptake (VO_2max) is accepted as an indicator of aerobic capacity, and some studies have shown that VO_2max increases with steroid use. The confounding factor is that tests of VO_2max are not necessarily good predictors of endurance performance.

However, anabolic steroids may have an indirect effect on aerobic capacity and endurance. It stands to reason that endurance athletes might benefit from steroids if they were then able to do more frequent, longer, and higher-intensity workouts as a result of drug use, as discussed in the previous chapter. In fact, a majority of athletes who use steroids say that they have experienced that benefit, but there is scant scientific evidence at present to buttress that claim.

Body Composition

Anabolic steroid users believe that using the drugs, in conjunction with training, will increase their lean body mass and decrease their fat mass. Whereas some researchers have reported no significant increases, others say there are increases. The reasons for these inconsistencies are in the study design and include factors such as how long the study lasted, the use of inexperienced subjects versus using trained athletes, steroid dosage, and so on. The consensus of experts is that steroids and a diet that is adequate for building muscle can contribute to increases in muscle mass beyond what could be achieved from training alone.

Strength Performance

Strength performance is another area where scientific steroid studies have contradictory findings. About half the research studies report no significant increase in strength with anabolic steroid use; the other half have reported a significant effect. However, individuals in these studies who are experienced in weight training and who continue training while taking anabolic steroids consistently experience increases in strength beyond those observed in control individuals from training alone. Additionally, the effects of high doses or prolonged use of anabolic steroids on body composition or strength have not been scientifically documented. Likewise, the residual effects of anabolic steroids on muscle mass or strength after termination of use have not been established.

Problems With Early Studies

When looking at the contradictory or inconsistent findings, people wonder why there aren't any simple yes or no answers. The scientific community was brought up short some years ago by the fact that numerous athletes were providing highly consistent accounts to indicate that steroids had a strong effect despite the inconsistent data from research. That prompted a number of scientists to take another look at the contradictory research data, and it soon became evident that something was wrong with the research.

In theory, there are several places where the research might have broken down. Briefly, the following factors can influence whether an improvement in athletic performance is seen with steroid use:

■ **Weight-training experience.** The early studies used a variety of subjects, from students enrolled in physical education classes to college athletes with a background in weight training. Considering just strength performance, it is easy to see how the weight training experience of the test subject could have a bearing. Inexperienced weight trainers make significant early strength gains when they begin weight-lifting programs regardless of whether they use steroids. These early gains likely would eclipse any steroid-induced gains. On the other hand, experienced weight trainers reach a plateau where further progress is difficult. In this select group of athletes, a small drug-assisted increase in strength would be very noticeable to the athlete and would be significantly greater than what could be achieved by training alone.

■ **Training intensity.** Some studies used low-intensity, short-duration, low-frequency workouts that are very unlike the high-intensity, long-duration, high-frequency workouts performed by athletes who are using anabolic steroids as a training aid.

■ **Dietary controls.** Many studies did not control dietary intake. The amount and proportion of carbohydrates, protein, and fat ingested in conjunction with steroids could significantly affect the degree of change in muscle mass, however.

■ **Drug dosage.** Athletes sometimes give themselves doses of anabolic steroids that are up to 100 times higher than normal replacement levels. None of the scientific studies have approached these dosage levels, nor could they because of the ethical constraints against giving high doses of drugs with known negative health consequences to healthy subjects. Moreover, athletes have been known to take drugs in sequences and combinations never duplicated in scientific studies.

■ **Specificity of training.** Some studies used a certain type of physical training, but the tests administered as a measure of efficacy were not based on the training that had been given. Training methods (isometric, isokinetic, and isotonic) stress muscles in different ways in order to develop them. Therefore, the difference between training and testing methods must surely affect the results.

NEW EVIDENCE OF STEROID EFFECTS

A study published in the *New England Journal of Medicine* in 1996 serves to put to rest most of the debate among scientists about whether steroids work (Bhasin et al., 1996). This study effectively controlled not only dietary factors, but also the type of exercise and the weight lifting experience of the subjects. Equally important, the dose of anabolic steroids that was administered exceeded the weekly amount taken by the average steroid user.

In this study, 43 men were randomly assigned to one of four groups: placebo with no strength training, testosterone ester with no strength training, placebo with strength training, and testosterone ester with strength training. The diet of all participants in the 10-week study was controlled. The men in the two groups receiving testosterone got 600 mg every week for 10 weeks, a dose that very likely exceeds the weekly amount taken by the many steroid users.

At the end of the 10 weeks, men who received testosterone but did no strength training gained significantly more muscle size and strength than those who received the placebo. The men who received both testosterone and strength training experienced increases in muscle size and strength that were far greater than those in the other three groups.

Note that until recently, the scientific literature addressed strength and body composition changes in men only. There had been no studies in women and children because of the ethical problems involved in giving masculinizing drugs whose effects in women and children are potentially irreversible. However, Franke and Berendonk (1997) have analyzed a number of classified documents saved after the collapse of the German Democratic Republic in 1990. From 1966 on, hundreds of athletes were treated with anabolic steroids each year, including minors of each sex. Anabolic steroids had a well-documented positive effect on athletic performance of adult women and children. However, it is reasonable to expect a positive effect on athletic performance of women and children from adding the male hormone testosterone (or one of its derivatives) because it is testosterone that is mainly responsible for muscular development in men.

Hormonal Side Effects for Women and Adolescent Boys

The answer to the question of whether anabolic steroids help women acquire more strength and power is yes. The downside is that women who add male hormones in the form of anabolic steroids can also expect to get many undesirable side effects, such as a deeper voice, loss of scalp hair, growth of facial hair, extension of pubic hair, and enlargement of the clitoris. These side effects were noted in a number of East German female athletes who were given anabolic steroids. These bodily alterations often remain after a woman stops taking steroids, and she will continue to have a somewhat masculinized appearance.

Young males on the threshold of puberty experience naturally rising androgen levels and more secretion of growth hormone. When anabolic steroids are taken in from an outside source, they can bring about a premature onset of these changes or alter the process. In addition to the well- known side effects of acne and breast development, high doses of steroids taken over a long period could lead to premature closure of the bony growth plates, causing diminished adult height. Also, increased aggressiveness could prove to be a negative matter at a time when emotions are easily roused by the normal process of adolescence.

ADDITIONAL STEROID DATA

The United States has had uncontrolled drug experimentation by athletes using steroids for about 40 years, and although this trial and error has undoubtedly produced "useful" anecdotal information on how to take steroids to improve athletic performance, the information is not in a form that can be easily surveyed or measured. Nor are the data available to other researchers who may want to see whether the study results can be reproduced. The scientific process of peer review, publication, and replication is how new medical knowledge is accumulated and tested.

One source of medically attended experiments with anabolic steroids has not yet been fully explored, however. In the former Eastern Bloc countries of Europe, sports drug experimentation was carried out under the sponsorship of the sports federations and with the help of physicians. A report on these sports "factories" and how they sponsored hormonal manipulations appeared in a 1992 issue of *U.S. News & World Report.* "Nothing demonstrated East Germany's indifference to the human cogs in its sports machine more than its unprecedented doping experiments on children," said the article, which went on to say that some 1,000 to 1,500 scientists, physicians, and trainers were involved in running controlled experiments on hundreds of athletes, some as young as age 14.

When the East German government fell, many of the classified records the government-sponsored, government-supported program of hormonal manipulation kept were destroyed. However, enough documents survived to provide clear evidence of the physical abuse of a generation of athletes. In a chilling article in *Clinical Chemistry* (Franke and Berendonk, 1997), two German authors detail some of the steroid experiments that were forced upon young East German athletes.

From 1972 through the early 1980s, the results of this systematized doping program were obvious; East Germany kept pace with the U.S. and the Soviet Union in the Olympic medal count, despite being a much smaller country. At the 1976 Olympic Games in Montreal, East German women swimmers won 11 out of 13 events.

The athletes themselves were sworn to secrecy. The pills and injections were called "vitamins" or "supporting therapy," and many young women were unaware that they were taking powerful hormones until they could no longer ignore the distressing changes in their bodies. Some female athletes even tried to drop sports, but were threatened with loss of financial support or expulsion from school.

The drug of choice was Oral-Turinabol, a steroid produced by the government pharmaceutical house. It may be that the worst aspect of this callous experimentation was the participation of physicians and other scientists in giving large doses of hormones to young athletes, and particularly to females. Most of the physicians were aware of the masculinizing effects of steroids, and some thought the program was unethical but were nevertheless subservient to the government, according to the authors.

These experiments were unethical and morally reprehensible, a type of experimentation that cannot be condoned, but researchers should study those data carefully, not only to chart the sports performance increases that could be ascribed to steroid use, but also to take careful note of negative outcomes and serious side effects. In that way, this medical literature of shame could bring a benefit to the world of sports.

INGREDIENTS OF ATHLETIC PERFORMANCE

In summary, we should be forthright in acknowledging that anabolic steroids work to enhance sports performance and allow most individuals to reach physical levels that they otherwise could never achieve. However, the message to young people should be that they can make significant gains in strength, muscle mass, and conditioning through hard work alone.

Moreover, we also must stress that superior athletic performance is a blend of several ingredients. John Lombardo, MD, the Ohio State University sports medicine physician who oversees the NFL drug program, has constructed a list of the elements that must be present to create peak sports performance. This list, which follows, makes it apparent that many systems must be operating right to achieve success:

■ **Level of conditioning.** Conditioning includes strength, flexibility, muscular endurance, and cardiovascular endurance. The importance of each of these differs, depending on the sport or event.

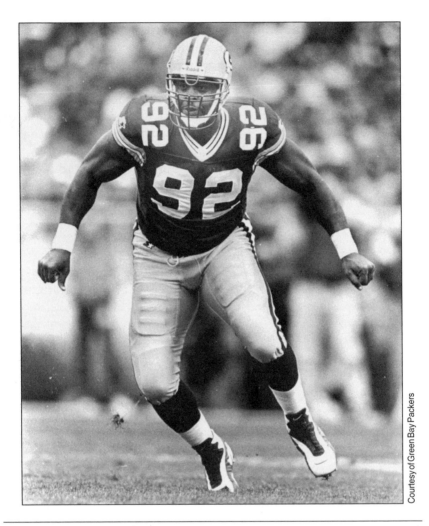

Great athletes like Reggie White develop from good genes, proper conditioning, superior skills, tough mindset, and good nutrition—drugs can't make up for poor conditioning or lack of skill.

Although steroids could have some impact on the level of conditioning, genetic heritage and the time and effort devoted to conditioning are probably much more important.

■ **Skill.** Genetic predisposition (talent) and repetition (practice) are the ingredients of skill, which is a learned behavior. Some sports require fine and complex motor skill development, whereas others may require only gross motor skill. There is no credible evidence that anabolic steroids can enhance skill.

■ **Diet.** The fuel the athlete needs for performance comes from his or her diet and, until recently, the role of nutrition has often been neglected. Consequently, many athletes have failed to maximize their muscle strength and conditioning gains by neglecting to maintain an adequate diet.

■ **Psyche.** The mental or psychological state of the athlete is usually described in such phrases as "having a game face on" or "getting up for a game," and these phrases refer to the proper mindset necessary for successful competition.

■ **Opponent.** How the opponent's style of play, strengths, and weaknesses compare to the athlete's.

■ **Arena.** The home-field advantage is a real phenomenon. Playing in familiar surroundings gives most athletes and teams an edge.

■ **Sleep.** Proper rest is necessary for the successful performance of any task, but it becomes even more critical in those requiring complex motor skills. Athletes sometimes have difficulty in resting properly before a contest because of anxiety or the new environment.

■ **Genes.** The athlete has no control over what very likely is the most important factor in sports success. Many of the characteristics that are necessary for a given sport are a result of genetic expression, which usually is referred to as talent or natural ability.

■ **Drugs.** Two effects can be seen with drugs. The use of drugs such as alcohol, marijuana, or cocaine before a sports contest can harm performance. Performance-enhancing drugs are those that are used to improve sports performance and that potentially can make a difference in the outcome of the competition.

COMMENTS BY DR. Y

Unfortunately, steroids do work and they work well. They help increase muscle mass and strength and permit an athlete to train more intensely, more often, and for longer periods of time. Is there a downside? You bet! Besides the fact that using steroids is cheating and against the law, these drugs can hurt you physically and psychologically. Although I believe that these reasons should be a sufficient deterrent to their use, some of my colleagues, with the best of intentions, have said that steroids do not work. Saying it doesn't make it so, and the result is a loss of credibility. Then when these same people speak of the very real adverse health effects, they often are not believed.

Still other colleagues argue that you can make the same gains without steroids; that it just takes longer. In my opinion that is wrong! High doses of steroids taken for long periods of time and combined with intensive strength training can result in muscle and strength gains that could never be achieved in a lifetime of hard work alone. Are there "freaks of nature," extraordinary physical specimens who are drug-free? Yes, but by definition they are rare, and certainly there are not enough of them to fill the rosters of the NFL, as the late Lyle Alzado noted. It is sad but true that anabolic steroids have the potential to take human capacities far beyond what can be done naturally. How tempting—but parents and coaches have to accept that fact and deal with it—and so do young athletes.

CHAPTER 4

HEALTH CONSEQUENCES OF STEROID USE

Most young steroid users are not thinking about whether they might harm their health. If anything, they consider themselves in better shape than their peers, and they focus on the benefits they believe steroids are giving them. Even with the best possible outcome, virtually all steroids users can expect to experience at least one negative health effect, however. If they are lucky, it may be something relatively minor like acne, loss of scalp hair, or temporary infertility. More serious consequences might be heart disease or a psychotic episode. Even more disturbing is the prospect of some as yet unknown consequence to either physical or mental health. A female or adolescent steroid user faces a longer list of known negative health effects, some of them permanent. The effects of steroid use on women are discussed separately later in this chapter because of the greater risks involved with such use.

The proven short-term side effects of steroid use are mostly reversible in men once they discontinue taking the drugs. Although at first glance this fact is cause for some optimism, most experts believe that too many users become psychologically dependent on steroids and continue using them; consequently, their adverse physical effects may not be reversed. Although very few users will be fortunate enough to experience no side effects, it is also true that only a few will experience the complete range of known short-term negative effects.

For several decades, scientists have stated that the long-term health effects of anabolic steroid use are unclear. Probably the long-term health effects will be related to the type of anabolic steroid, dose, frequency of use, age of initiation, and concurrent drug use. None of this has been examined through epidemiologic studies. And the fact that some individuals use large doses of anabolic steroids for prolonged periods of time whereas others use therapeutic doses intermittently further complicates the process of determining long-term health effects.

We can expect some new data to emerge within the next decade, simply because the pool of older users and former users is growing and aging. What we can say with some certainty now is that there are clear risks that increase with higher dosages and longer usage.

PHYSICAL EFFECTS

Putting the risks of steroids into a single list so that very diverse actions are side by side and out of context is a gross oversimplification, but such a list is easier for the reader. (Please consult the list of recommended readings at the end of the book for a more detailed discussion of health risks.)

The undesirable physical health consequences that are most often associated with abuse of anabolic steroids include the following:

- Cosmetic changes
- Musculoskeletal injuries
- Infertility
- Heart disease
- Stroke
- Prostate problems
- Liver toxicity

Physical Appearance

Oily skin and acne, which can cause scarring, are among the most frequently observed side effects of steroid use among athletes. Another is changes in hair patterns, such as increased body hair growth and an acceleration in male pattern baldness in those predisposed to it. Breast enlargement (gynecomastia) in men or shrinkage of breast tissue in women are side effects considered by most to be unwanted.

Many of these effects are permanent and, not surprisingly, distressing to the individual, although none is considered a serious risk to life or limb. The most serious threat to appearance is the very real possibility that chronic steroid use, especially prior to puberty or in early adolescence, could cause the premature closure of the growth plates of the long bones so that adult stature is significantly shorter than nature intended.

Muscle and Bone Injuries

So far, the musculoskeletal injuries sustained by steroid users cannot be distinguished from those seen in strength athletes with extraordinary muscle development who do not use steroids. Animal studies suggest that the risk of tendon rupture may be increased in steroid users, however. There are several anecdotal reports of injuries in athletes whose muscle mass exceeded the strength of the attachment to bone. The most common type of injury that athletes sustain is damage to the ligaments and tendons.

Infertility

The reversible effect of steroid administration on male fertility has been studied for more than 20 years with a thought to using anabolic steroids as a male contraceptive. Taking synthetic sex hormones disrupts the normal hormonal process. Many steroid users report an increase in libido initially, but diminished sex drive is associated with prolonged use. Most men who self-administer high doses of steroids become infertile during the period of use and for some time afterwards, perhaps six months or more. Infertility cannot be reliably produced in all males, and not all steroids are equally effective. Several researchers believe there is a risk of sterility with prolonged use at high dosage levels, but no case has ever been reliably documented. A common problem related to the infertility issue is a significant reduction in the size of the testicles as a result of steroid use.

Heart Disease

There are good reasons to believe that long-term abuse of anabolic steroids increases the incidence of heart disease, even though that fact has not yet been demonstrated unequivocally. Several known bodily changes in steroid users could explain this possible increased risk of heart disease.

Lipid Levels

The use of anabolic steroids causes a reduction in the serum level of a type of blood fat known as HDLC (high-density lipoprotein cholesterol), probably because the steroids stimulate a liver enzyme that regulates fats in the blood. This reduction of the so-called "good cholesterol" is clinically significant and has been identified as a major risk factor for heart disease and stroke in epidemiological studies of men who are not steroid users. This reduction appears to be reversible; HDLC levels begin to recover within about a month after steroid use is discontinued.

Although this depression of HDLC has been documented in a number of studies of athletes taking steroids, it's not an inevitable consequence because not all steroids produce the effect to the same extent. Oral steroids have a significantly more pronounced negative impact on HDLC levels, probably because of their overall stressful impact upon the liver. A few studies have reported an increase in total cholesterol, but most do not. It appears that the decrease in circulating HDLC is offset by an increase in low-density lipoprotein cholesterol (LDLC) so that the total cholesterol level remains the same.

Glucose Tolerance

Some anabolic steroids can cause glucose intolerance which, like blood fat changes, is considered a risk factor for heart disease in itself. These steroids can also impair the body's mechanism for regulating the amount of insulin so that too much is produced. Researchers have suggested that testosterone and steroids increase the risk of heart disease through an effect on insulin.

Blood Pressure

There have been claims that steroids cause high blood pressure, but this claim appears to be exaggerated, based on a few studies that demonstrated increases in blood pressure that were of little or no clinical significance.

Heart Tissue

The effects of testosterone on the heart muscle of animals were first described more than 60 years ago, and evidence that anabolic steroids alter myocardial performance in animals was presented more than 40 years ago. These animal studies showed that the heart has androgen receptors and that anabolic steroids can cause cardiac dysfunction.

Enlargement of the heart (*cardiomegaly*) is not always a bad thing. Exercise itself causes an increase in heart size that is not dangerous but represents a physical adaptation by the heart muscle to increase the blood supply to meet increased physical demands. With each beat of a normal heart, the main pumping chamber (left ventricle) ejects between 50 and 80 percent of the blood in the chamber, depending on the activity level. This is called the ejection fraction. When the heart becomes larger because of disease or drug use, its efficiency diminishes; the ejection fraction may fall below 40 percent, which means that the heart pump is no longer efficient. When this happens, the individual will have fatigue and shortness of breath and be unable to sustain a high level of physical activity.

In 1988, the first case of cardiomyopathy (a medical term referring to heart disease) and stroke (cerebrovascular accident) associated with anabolic steroids was reported. Since then, other case reports have indicated that using anabolic steroids can cause this unhealthy enlargement and weakening of the main pumping chamber.

Steve Courson, a former pro football player who acknowledged steroid use during his career (see chapter 1), was diagnosed with a dilated cardiomyopathy, meaning that his heart had enlarged in an unhealthy way and lost its capacity to pump efficiently. A prudent person might conclude that this enlargement was a long-term steroid effect. What confounds the situation is that Steve admits he also abused alcohol during that period of his life, and alcohol is a well-documented risk factor for this type of heart disease. These not uncommon life situations make it difficult for researchers to completely separate the various risks and identify a single causative factor.

An autopsy of a steroid-using athlete who died in his early twenties showed that extensive areas of heart muscle had been replaced with fibrous tissue. His death could have been caused by a viral infection or an infection of the lining of the heart, however. We cannot say with absolute certainty that steroids caused his death. Many experts do believe that there is potential for damage to the heart tissue, however. It is likely that there is an increased incidence of disease to the heart muscle among athletes who use anabolic steroids, but an unequivocal causal relationship is unlikely to be established until a properly designed epidemiological study provides careful control of other risk factors.

Stroke and Heart Attack

Steroid abuse has emerged as a possible cause of thrombotic stroke, the kind caused by a blood clot. The medical literature contains several case reports of athletes and one of a young man who secretly increased his intake of a form of testosterone that had been pre-scribed to help him mature (a legitimate use of the drug) that had this kind of stroke. In addition, several cases of stroke have been reported in Japanese men who received large doses of anabolic steroids as treatment for a type of anemia. Although no direct evidence exists, the clinical circumstances of these case reports is suspicious and suggests a possible relationship between steroid use and the risk of stroke. If a causal relationship does exist, it could represent the first evidence that steroids have potentially life-threatening short-term effects.

Prostate Diseases

Women who take oral contraceptives, which also are sex hormones, have a slightly greater risk of breast cancer. The parallel in men may be a higher risk of prostate cancer as a result of taking steroids. Although it usually is a disease of older men, prostate cancer is the second leading cause of cancer death (after lung cancer) in American men. If steroids increase the risk, it is a matter of serious concern. Physicians know that prostate cancer is negatively affected by the male hormone testosterone; standard treatment for this disease already includes reducing or blocking testosterone within the body. One case report describes a bodybuilder who had prostate cancer at the early age of 40 years. It is quite possible that today's steroid abusers will face a higher risk for prostate cancer as they age.

Liver Disease and Cancer

Steroids definitely have a strong negative effect on liver function, which is not surprising because the liver is the principal site where steroids are cleared from the body. Virtually all changes in the structure of the liver have been associated with the use of a type of oral steroids known as 17 alpha-alkylated steroids. When steroids are taken by mouth, the liver is exposed to the full dose of the drug before it is distributed in the circulation. This exposure can be particularly dangerous in individuals who already have poor liver function from other causes. Anabolic steroid abuse can harm the liver in several ways.

Jaundice

Blockage of the bile flow, which causes jaundice (yellowing of the skin and the whites of the eyes), has been seen in patients with serious diseases who are being treated with anabolic steroids. The first suggestion that some anabolic steroids might cause liver problems came when physicians tried to use methyltestosterone (an anabolic steroid) to treat the severe itching associated with obstructive jaundice. Most patients with jaundice got worse. Although athletes have used steroids that have been associated with bile flow blockage and jaundice, most probably stop taking steroids when jaundice occurs. For these reasons and the fact there have been only a few documented clinical cases of jaundice in athletes, almost no information exists about this condition in healthy individuals.

Peliosis Hepatis

Peliosis hepatis is a potentially life-threatening condition in which blood-filled cysts develop in the liver. Before the development of steroids, this condition was seen almost exclusively in patients with pulmonary tuberculosis. Now, more than 70 cases of peliosis have been reported in association with intake of male hormones. The reason that this condition is so dangerous is that it is not easily diagnosed and patients often have no symptoms. If the cysts rupture, the patient can die, with little or no warning, from internal hemorrhage.

Liver Tumors

Taking anabolic steroids increases the risk of liver tumors. The type of tumor seen most often behaves more like a noncancerous, or benign, type of liver tumor. These benign tumors can still be life threatening, however. At least several of the steroid-related tumors were diagnosed because the tumors ruptured and caused serious or fatal internal bleeding. There is one report of a hepatocellular carcinoma in a steroid-using athlete who died from this metastatic cancer. Another athlete who used steroids died from internal hemorrhage after a type of tumor called an adenoma ruptured. A third patient also had an adenoma but survived after it was removed surgically.

The occurrence of anabolic steroid-related liver tumors appears to be considerably higher than the rate of liver tumors associated with oral contraceptive use by women. Liver tumors are rare among the estimated 30 million women in the United States who take oral contraceptives; fewer than 400 cases have been reported in women since 1937. Moreover, 92 percent of the first cases reported after oral contraceptives became widely used were benign. Although the prevalence of anabolic steroid use is nowhere near that of oral contraceptives, the literature already documents nearly 100 cases of steroid-associated liver tumors. Therefore, the risk of harm to the liver is substantial.

PSYCHOLOGICAL EFFECTS

So much attention was given to the serious physical health consequences of anabolic steroid use that it was some time before researchers realized that the psychological and behavioral effects might be equally important. Anabolic steroids were used from the late 1930s until the mid-1980s as an accepted and seemingly successful treatment for mood and mental disorders, including psychosis and depression. The psychological effects of giving therapeutic dosages of anabolic steroids in clinical settings include an increase in mental alertness, mood elevation, improvements in memory and concentration, and reduction of fatigue sensations.

Other research has shown that testosterone has a significant effect on both the development and function of the nervous system. It appears that the effect of testosterone/anabolic steroids on brain function results in an elevation of norepinephrine (nature's version of adrenaline) levels in the brain. Anabolic steroids also have been shown to elicit changes in brain activity similar to those seen with amphetamines and tricyclic antidepressants.

Increased Aggression

The relationship between natural testosterone levels and dominance and aggressive behavior in various species of animals is well known. Of course, as we move up the evolutionary scale, social learning plays a significantly greater role in behavior. Although the relationship between testosterone and aggression is quite pronounced in mice and rats, the association is somewhat less consistent in monkeys, apes, and especially man. Nevertheless, a number of studies have looked at naturally occurring testosterone levels in men, and many, but not all, have shown an association between elevated testosterone levels and increases in both subjectively perceived aggressive behavior and observed aggressive behavior.

During the past decade, case reports of individual steroid users have suggested that mood swings and psychotic episodes, some of violent proportions, may be associated with steroid use in particular individuals. This association is in contrast to earlier clinical findings. In several of these cases that came to trial, the defendants alleged that

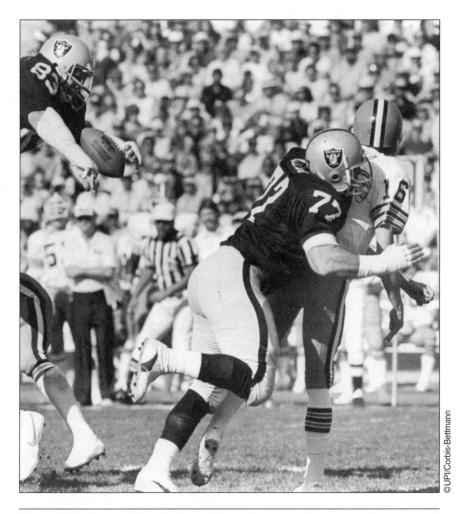

©UPI/Corbis-Bettmann

The late Lyle Alzado (77) and other acknowledged steroid users have demonstrated behaviors that some have referred to as "roid rage."

the presumed psychological and behavioral effects of anabolic ster-oids significantly influenced the commission of criminal acts. Re-cently, data from a nationwide study confirmed prior studies and demonstrated a strong association between anabolic steroid use and self-acknowledged acts of violence against people and crimes against property (Yesalis et al. 1993; see chapter 1).

Although most scientists apparently agree that anabolic ster-oids, especially at high doses, seem to increase aggressiveness, not all studies reached this conclusion. Although three prospective, blinded studies documenting aggression or adverse overt behavior resulting from steroid use have been reported, two recent clinical trials, in which fairly substantial doses of steroids were administered to volunteers over a period of weeks, didn't detect any widespread demonstrable sexual or psychological effects.

One matter of particular debate among scientists and users alike is whether the condition popularly known as "roid rage" exists. "Roid rage" is a descriptive term for spontaneous, highly aggressive, out-of-control behavior where the police either were called or should have intervened. Some scientists and users claim they have observed steroid-induced fits of reckless or even criminal behavior, but others question the existence of these episodes, their frequency, or whether steroids were the cause of the observed behavior. If this phenomenon is real, it is relatively rare (probably less than 1 percent) among steroid users. Even among those affected, the impact of previous mental illness or abuse of other drugs is still unclear. Moreover, the placebo effect may play a role in that so much media attention has been directed toward steroid-induced aggression that users may be experiencing a self-fulfilling prophecy.

User Dependence

Another intriguing question is whether the potential exists for physi-cal dependence on anabolic steroids. Although only one case study purportedly has demonstrated physical addiction, several studies have demonstrated behavior, perceptions, and attitudes in some steroid users (25 percent to more than 50 percent) that are indicative of psychological dependence. Despite this finding, user characteris-tics that might be predictors of dependence are poorly understood.

Overall, the behavioral effects of anabolic steroids are variable, transient upon discontinuation of the drugs, and appear to be related to the type, and possibly the dosage, of anabolic steroids. Moreover, with an estimated 1 million or more past or current users in the United States, only an extremely small percentage of individuals using anabolic steroids appear to have experienced mental disturbances severe enough to need clinical treatment.

WOMEN AND STEROIDS

The effort in the United States over the past 20 years to place women's sports on a par with men's sports has served to let more athletically talented women play sports at the collegiate, national, and international levels. Because the competition has grown fiercer and the rewards are greater, however, adolescent girls and young women now face some of the same pressures to use drugs as males.

Masculinizing Effects

Women who take anabolic steroids face extra hazards in that they are taking male sex hormones that will change their bodies and make them more masculine. Most of the physical differences between men and women are due to higher levels of testosterone in men. Women secrete a sexual hormone called estrogen that affects fat distribution and the shape of the pelvis. They do have small amounts of circulating natural testosterone, and the adrenal glands or ovaries also secrete some other androgens (male hormones).

When the balance is altered by taking male sex hormones (steroids) from outside the body, women quickly see masculinizing side effects like loss of scalp hair, growth of facial hair, spread of pubic hair, deepening of the voice, and enlargement of the clitoris—effects that are mostly permanent. Acne is likely. Women will experience the same, mostly reversible effects on cholesterol and liver enzyme function as men. Increased aggression also has been observed.

Estimated Use by Women

The prospect of going bald and growing a beard is enough to deter many women from steroid use, but it doesn't deter everyone. Steroid use by adolescent girls in the United States is low but significant. An estimated .5 to 2 percent or more of high school senior girls have used anabolic steroids, and some began as early as the sixth grade. The highest female steroid use is believed to be among women who engage in bodybuilding, power lifting, and other sports that call for strength.

When female collegiate athletes were asked to estimate the level of steroid use among competitors in their own sport, they judged that 5 percent of swimmers, 6 percent of basketball players, and 10 percent of track and field athletes had used steroids within the past year. A fourth of the participants in softball, tennis, gymnastics, field hockey, volleyball, and lacrosse believed there had been some steroid use in their sports within the previous 12 months. Positive drug tests in women athletes have been reported in the sports of power lifting, bodybuilding, the shot put, javelin throw, swimming, cycling, and running.

In light of the known negative consequences, researchers have been keenly interested in examining the reasons women use steroids. Richard Strauss, MD, editor-in-chief of *The Physician and Sportsmedicine* and a faculty member at the Ohio State University Medical Center, has a special interest in identifying the factors that move women to take steroids. In 1985, he did in-depth interviews with 10 female users who took steroids in cycles, just as men do. (Dr. Strauss did not prescribe or supply their drugs.) Their comments were revealing. Although most women view the masculinizing side effects of steroids as undesirable, these effects were acceptable to these female steroid users and their partners as the price for the gains they reported in muscle strength, muscle size, and sports performance.

The 10 women Dr. Strauss studied took both oral and injectable drugs. Two of the products were veterinary drugs. One of the women took a moderate amount of a single drug, but another took five different anabolic steroids stacked during a 10-week use cycle, a regimen that would be considered moderately heavy use in a man. Dr. Strauss reported that the women justified their steroid use on the grounds that steroids were necessary for them to win and also because they felt it was within their individual rights to use steroids as they wished.

All 10 women reported significant increases in muscle strength and size and enhanced sports performance. All 10 women had lower voices, and seven said this effect was undesirable. Five women noted a decrease in breast size; four attached no significance to this change, and one thought the decrease was desirable. Nine had increased facial hair, eight had clitoral enlargement, and six noticed an increase in sexual desire. Cessation of menstruation or lighter flow was common. Eight women reported increased aggressiveness. Six of them felt this effect was desirable because it enhanced their drive to compete; others found that aggressiveness caused problems in interpersonal relationships. (Some of the women reported that their steroid-induced aggressiveness created friction with family members and associates.)

Additional Effects

In addition to the masculinizing effects that a female user will definitely notice, other changes are occurring that may go undetected. Some women believe that menopause may be reached sooner in women who have taken steroids for a long time. There have been scattered reports in Europe of birth defects in the infants of female athletes who took steroids and accounts of difficulty with conception. Polycystic ovaries have been reported in some transsexual individuals being treated with male sex hormones for a long time.

Although women, regardless of sport, are generally thought to use lower dosages of anabolic steroids than men, the amount they do use is quite enough to cause damage. If a man who normally produces about 7 milligrams a day of natural testosterone takes 100 milligrams of steroids daily, he exposes himself to a 10- to 15-fold increase in testosterone. On the other hand, a woman who normally produces .3 milligrams a day and takes 100 milligrams of steroids a day exposes herself to more than a 300-fold increase in testosterone beyond the normal level for women!

Another interesting aspect of female steroid use is that some women who have undergone masculinizing changes exhibit denial about these changes; they appear to have the same lack of perception about their true body image as do women who are anorexic. One of the guests on a national television program on steroids was a heavily muscled and masculinized steroid-taking female bodybuilder who looked like a cross dresser in an extremely feminine sundress. As the studio audience viewed a pre-steroid photograph of her on a monitor, they jeered and laughed when she insisted she represented the "new ideal of feminine beauty."

A LOOK AT WOMEN'S SPORTS

The good news about women's sports is that they are finally getting some of the same recognition as men's sports. The bad news is that they now have many of the same problems, including drug use. "Women are headed down the same bad path as the men," sighs Rene Portland, head women's basketball coach at Pennsylvania State University. "The 'winning at all costs' mentality, cutting corners, kids not making their own choices and decisions—women's sports has it all."

Portland is enthusiastic about women participating in sports, and she agrees with Miami Heat basketball coach Pat Riley that teamwork is the essence of life, saying that being on a team "helps you be part of the team in a family or at a future job. It teaches time management skills, and it improves self-confidence." The problem comes, she says, when the athlete's aim is transferred from the sport itself to the sport as a means to an end—to money, a college scholarship, popularity, or national recognition. When the emphasis is on winning, and the pressure is unremitting, women are vulnerable to using anabolic steroids and other drugs to enhance their sports performance, even at the cost of their health.

Portland says that having more scholarships in women's athletics in the United States has been positive in the main, although some coaches now expect more than is reasonable from female scholarship athletes. "Some (women's) coaches are flat out nuts," she asserts. "I've seen screaming, riding the kids, unbelievable behavior. We've lost the reality of the positive side of sports in many cases." Parents come in for criticism too. Portland said parental pressure can be extreme and that a young woman who calls home about a sports-related problem often is told to "gut it out," whether that means playing with an injury or submitting to harsh treatment. Some young women may see performance-enhancing drugs as a way to relieve the pressure.

This coach doesn't believe in demeaning any of the young women who play for her, nor does she insist that basketball is all important, all the time. "Coaches and parents cannot be naïve to the pressures that are put on kids that will cause them to look to the outside for help to meet our expectations," says Portland. Her remarks about the proper role of basketball may seem odd coming from a woman who played college basketball at top-ranked Immaculata and who has guided the Lady Lions basketball team to new heights of popularity. A crowd of about 200 for a women's basketball game was about the norm when she arrived at Penn State. Now they play in front of about 5,000 per game.

She doesn't think that steroids are rampant in women's collegiate basketball, and Portland tells her Lady Lions frankly to forget drugs. She has high praise for the Penn State Freshman Experience Program, which deals extensively with preventing drug use. As for the perks and privileges that can cause some athletes to turn to drugs to keep up, Portland doesn't cater to that either. "Kids don't need 200 pairs of sneakers a year," she says. "Lots of people have won in canvas shoes. We shouldn't teach them that everything has to be perfect in order for them to succeed because many times, things won't go perfectly in real life."

She is secretly proud when former players swear their most trying business problems are hardly worth mentioning after playing basketball for Rene Portland. A woman with a husband, three children, and family responsibilities in addition to her job as head coach, Portland preaches balance in addition to hard work, responsibility, and time management skills. In her view, a balanced approach may be the most effective method of countering pressures and temptations as women's sports continue to grow. Many of the worst steroid problems with female athletes have arisen within systems where the coach and/or sports organization is all-powerful and the athlete has little voice. Portland likes for her athletes to take control of their careers, as well as their sport.

STEROID RISK

In summary, the short-term physical effects of anabolic steroids are well-documented. Some are benign and temporary, but others could pose a significant threat to long-term health, especially if the associated risk factors (such as low HDLC levels) are sustained for long periods of time. This possibility is real because some steroid users become psychologically dependent on these drugs. The usual process, when that happens, is a significant prolongation of steroid-taking, which also prolongs the time of increased risk for consequent diseases.

Psychological dependence aside, much less agreement exists on the impact of these hormones on the development of psychiatric conditions that are serious enough to warrant professional care. The long-term health consequences of anabolic steroids have not been investigated and are unclear at this time. The sober bottom line, taking everything into account, is that any athlete, male or female, would be foolish to conclude that using anabolic steroids is without consequences.

PREVENTING AND TREATING STEROID USE

PART II

The methods that have been devised to stop steroid use can be divided into those that detect use, punish users, educate potential users about the dangers, and help current users stop. The chapters in Part II deal with these methods, which should be used together for best results. No one method alone will be successful.

There can be no doubt that one of the most effective lines of defense against drugs at the high school and even collegiate levels is the attitude of the parents and coaches. A parent or coach who pushes winning at all costs may not realize how much psychological pressure is transferred to the athletes. Drug testing has become a fact of life at most colleges and at a handful of high schools. Although it is undoubtedly a deterrent, there are fewer drug users to catch with drug tests when the coach has a personal drug-free philosophy.

University of Iowa wrestling coach Dan Gable says that he talks frankly with his wrestlers about anabolic steroids. As an Olympic gold medalist himself, Gable knows first-hand the pressures on elite athletes. "There is more to being a winner now," he acknowledges, saying that there is more temptation because of the financial rewards, the lucrative professional contracts, and the media attention. Gable believes that the steroid problem in wrestling is not as bad as it is in some sports, and adds that he "jumps on any drug use really hard."

67

In his words, "Besides the health effects, what you lose when you use steroids is mental toughness. The key to victory is that the strongest mind wins," he explains. "You can get physical strength with steroids, but you lose the mental toughness it took to get to a high level naturally. You get mental toughness through really brutal hard work." Steroids, he concludes, hurt mental toughness by serving as a crutch.

The Iowa wrestlers have a program that incorporates random testing, along with education and supervision. Gable agrees that education is a potentially strong line of defense, especially when combined with drug testing, but he also recognizes that the downside of some educational programs is that they increase the level of awareness about steroids and may make them seem attractive to an athlete who had not considered using them. To avoid this paradoxical effect, any education programs must be carefully structured and tested.

In addition to drug testing and prevention, there are regulatory efforts to control steroids. When steroid use is detected in sports, sanctions may be imposed, which usually means loss of the right to compete. When steroid use is paired with out-of-bounds behavior, the penalty could be loss of freedom if laws are broken. Both state and federal laws control steroid prescription and sales, and black market steroid dealers face criminal penalties as do crack or heroin sellers.

Unfortunately, sales continue to flourish. The Drug Enforcement Agency estimates that anabolic steroids represent a 400 million-dollar black market in this country alone. Enforcement of steroid laws already on the books has lagged because of lack of manpower and money, as well as lenient federal sentencing guidelines. With the current upswing in the cycle of recreational drug use, it is unlikely that the government will target steroid users for enforcement action, with perhaps the exception of dealers who handle very large quantities.

Still another way to combat steroid use is to treat it medically. With most other illicit drugs, society has moved away from simply punishing users toward the medical treatment model that views some drug use as an illness or an addiction. Experts do not believe that anabolic steroids are physically addictive in themselves, but most recognize that a significant number of users will become psychologically dependent on these drugs and some of those will not be able to stop using steroids without professional help. However, not many mental health professionals have experience in dealing with steroid users, and fewer still are being trained to deal with steroid abusers. The implications of this lack of experienced personnel are unknown at this time, but they could mean that some users will not be able to get the help they need to quit.

A strong index of suspicion can serve as still another line of defense. Ask questions. Be informed. A former football lineman remarked casually on a sports radio program in Chicago that it was hard to compare the top linemen of his era with today's linemen because of their size. A player weighing more than 250 pounds was rare in his day. He and the host then named a number of current linemen who weigh in excess of 300 pounds. Not once did they mention how this great increase in size might have come about. One objective of this book is to raise awareness about body development. In truth, it is very difficult to naturally pack 300 pounds of mostly lean body mass on a human frame. Fat, yes; lean body mass, no.

Some athletes are cheating and getting away with it. Public sentiment for stopping the use of steroids and other performance-enhancing drugs at the elite level is not particularly high. In all likelihood, this is because it is sometimes hard to see the victims. Moreover, many Americans are entertained by watching bigger-than-life athletes perform superhuman feats. This seeming indifference is in keeping with what we know about drug use in American society. However, sports are an integral part of American society. Because they have value for all of us, we must all bear some responsibility for helping find a solution to the problem of steroid abuse.

CHAPTER 5

DRUG TESTING

Drug testing is the method that has been chosen to identify those athletes who use banned drugs to enhance their sports performance at the expense of the athletes who don't take drugs. It has become clear that drug testing alone will not be enough to stop steroid use. While drug testing is the first line of defense at the collegiate, Olympic, and professional levels of sport, athletes, coaches and trainers, and parents must shoulder the responsibility for keeping the playing field level at the junior high and high school levels.

Two decades have passed since sports drug testing became part of the Olympic Games. Drug testing is now part of professional sports, collegiate sports, and to a very small extent, high school sports. The technology of drug testing has made significant advances; cheating methods have also evolved and grown more sophisticated.

Drug testing is an extremely complex subject that evokes strong opinions. For that reason, this book contains two chapters on drug testing. This chapter covers the development of drug testing and the procedures that are used. Chapter 11, "Troubles With Drug Testing," deals with the problems related to drug testing and how political issues play a role in how drug testing is performed.

HISTORY OF DRUG TESTING

The desire to gain a competitive edge probably dates back to the first foot races organized by prehistoric humans. Human nature being what it is, we can safely assume that athletes have always looked for ways to enhance physical performance. Nothing is inherently wrong with this concept so long as the contest is carried out on a level playing field. Some practices that any athlete can do and that do not pose a significant health risk have been shown to enhance performance. Strength training, mental readiness exercises, affirmations, changing locations or practice habits, and diet are just a few of the options that are open to anyone who wants to give them a try. When an athlete is willing to break the rules to win, the playing field is no longer level.

When society first became concerned about drugs and sports, horses were the subject. The Austrian Jockey Club summoned a Russian chemist to Vienna in 1910 to see whether he could detect the presence of alkaloids in the saliva of racehorses, and the idea of testing racehorses was born. Given the vast amounts of money associated with horse racing, those in the sport believed testing was prudent to make sure that horses were competing only on their own merits and without the aid of drugs. The chief objection to horse doping is, of course, exactly the same objection that arises in human contests: the presence of drugs renders the contest unfair.

Until the advent of modern chemistry, the performance enhancement choices for athletes were pretty much limited to using potions, lotions, tinctures, herbal extracts, and other substances that were ingested or rubbed on the body. The very earliest instances of human doping for sports performance enhancement is lost to history, but it appears that it was neither well-organized nor highly effective until the advent of amphetamines, one of the first drugs that could make a difference in athletic contests.

European sports circles of the 1950s were gravely concerned about cyclists and soccer players who were taking amphetamines. This drug war was already well underway in 1960, but it first came to public attention after a Danish cyclist died during the Summer Olympic Games in Rome, a death that was later linked to amphetamine abuse. Track athlete Dick Howard died the same year after using "pep pills."

Then British cyclist Tommy Simpson died in the French Alps during the 1967 Tour de France. As Simpson struggled up the

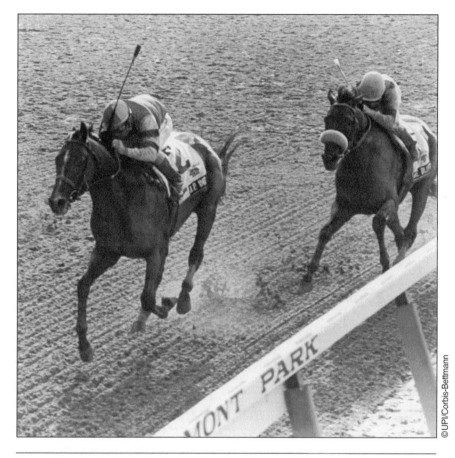

Drug use in sport first gained media attention in conjunction with horse racing in the early 1900s.

mountain in the blazing sun, spectators could see he was in trouble. The champion cyclist finally reeled across the road and fell from his bike but he waved off assistance and managed to remount. This time, he traveled only a short distance before going down for good. The amphetamines found in his body and in his pockets had allowed him to continue well past the point of physical exhaustion.

By the time the public was alerted, amphetamines had already become a staple in endurance sports. Many former baseball and football players recall a time when they were distributed like candy. Unlike steroids, amphetamines were also widely used by the general public for their usefulness in staving off fatigue and in dieting. Therefore, when the dangers of amphetamines, including addiction and even sudden death, became known, many people had experienced the seductive appeal of "pep pills" for themselves. The ensuing outcry stimulated some sports organizations and legislative bodies to institute drug testing of athletes and to pass legislation to regulate drug use.

Concern about amphetamines was one of the first issues for the emerging specialty of sports medicine to confront. Various sports and medical groups held symposia from the 1950s onward to discuss the drug-related issues. Doping was the main topic of discussion when the International Sports Medicine Congress met in Paris in 1959.

Meanwhile, with amphetamines assuming a high profile, little notice was paid to steroids, which were quietly sweeping through the athlete ranks by the mid 1960s. A harbinger of the future were Eastern bloc female athletes who looked suspiciously like men. In the United States, the sport of football took on a completely new appearance as ever larger and stronger linemen became the norm. In the 1960s and 1970s, the team physician, who also monitored athletes for side effects, commonly prescribed steroids. Very little thought was given to the ethical aspects of steroid use at that time. Moreover, the scientific community was not in agreement on whether steroids built lean muscle mass and increased strength.

Drug Testing of Banned Substances

The first really scientific drug testing came about in the 1960s because the techniques of analytical chemistry, especially the use of the gas chromatograph, had become sufficiently refined to detect more and more doping agents or their metabolites in biological fluids, chiefly urine. The work of setting up procedures and tests for drug testing was pioneered by Dr. Arnold Beckett of London, England, one of the original members of the IOC Medical Commission. The first official list of banned substances was drawn up in 1963 and included narcotics, amine stimulants, alkaloids, and all analeptic agents, respiratory tonics, and certain hormones. Simply achieving agreement on a list of substances to be banned was a major hurdle because of the differences of personality, point of view, and national interest involved among the participants.

Prince Alexandre De Merode of Belgium had become aware of the doping problems in his own sport of cycling and stepped in to work with the newly formed Medical Commission. By the end of 1967, the

IOC had drafted rules prohibiting doping. Although drug testing officially began with random testing during the 1968 Olympic Winter Games, that testing was a far cry from the sophisticated process of today.

One of the most important international figures in drug testing was Dr. Manfred Donike who, until his death in August 1995, was director of the Institute for Biochemistry Laboratory in Cologne, Germany. Dr. Donike brought the zeal of a detective to the art of drug testing and was influential in setting standards for drug testing laboratories and in refining technology. He was in charge of drug testing for the 1972 Olympic Games in Munich.

In 1980, the IOC drafted its own requirements for accreditation that would apply to drug testing laboratories. These standards are stringent so far as technical and professional competence go. The first IOC-approved drug testing laboratory in the United States was the Paul Ziffren Olympic Analytical Facility at the University of California at Los Angeles, which handled the testing for the Los Angeles Summer Olympic Games of 1984. The director of that laboratory is Dr. Don Catlin, who also is a member of the IOC Medical Commission. The second laboratory was set up at Indiana University and ran the drug testing for the Pan American Games in 1987 under the direction of Dr. John Baenziger.

Both laboratories are part of a worldwide network of approximately 25 laboratories. In addition to the two in the United States, there is one in Montreal, Canada and one each in China, Korea, Australia, Japan, and South Africa. The rest are in Europe. According to Dr. Catlin, laboratories are being developed in Hungary, Poland, Malaysia, Puerto Rico, Brazil, Zimbabwe, Indonesia, and Turkey. For the 1996 Olympic Games, temporary accreditation was granted to a drug testing laboratory of Smith, Kline & Beecham in Atlanta. Under an agreement with UCLA, approximately 30 staff members from that lab assumed responsibility for the steroid testing at the Games.

The IOC has its own complicated testing protocols and, additionally, its laboratories are forbidden to test samples unless they are submitted from a bona fide sports program. This restriction is to prevent athletes from using laboratory facilities to find out how to evade detection. Drug testers themselves concede that differences exist in laboratory performance. The ability to detect doping agents is only one aspect of performance. Other important yardsticks of a laboratory's work are analysis capacity and turnover rate between the time samples are received and results are reported.

For instance, during the Olympic Games of 1972 in Munich, more than 2,000 samples were analyzed within the 14 days of the competition, which was a large task carried out in a brief period of time. With the increase in the number of athletes participating in international sports, the workload of the testing laboratories has also increased. In Atlanta, some 1,850 samples were tested, which was very difficult because of the new high-resolution mass spectrometer machines being used.

Dr. Baenziger observed that the two IOC-accredited U.S. laboratories are the only two in the entire IOC network that routinely go through published proficiency testing. This difference does not mean, he notes, that they are the only ones doing excellent work. It is hard to compare laboratories in different countries, however. Procedures and equipment may vary slightly. Relatively well-funded operations like Dr. Catlin's lab at UCLA or Dr. Baenziger's lab in Indianapolis have more resources than most and enjoy a reputation for high-quality work.

Even if great care is taken in handling the specimens and in doing the laboratory work, the economic and political conditions in various countries most certainly affect the operations of an IOC-accredited drug testing laboratory, although the extent of this effect on false positive or false negative tests has never been publicly documented. For example, the IOC-accredited laboratory in what was East Germany played a major role in assisting its athletes in circumventing drug tests.

There has been much speculation about whether the Chinese laboratory has acted in a similar fashion. This concern received widespread publicity after Chinese women made extraordinary strides in world class competition, both in swimming and in track. After some of them were identified as steroid users through drug tests at international competitions in 1993 and 1994, the Chinese sports programs came under close scrutiny.

One of drug testing's finest moments came during the 1983 Pan American Games in Caracas, Venezuela, when Dr. Donike arrived unannounced and promptly demonstrated that the drug testing technology was up to the challenge of the day. Although only 12 athletes lost medals because of positive steroid tests, the airport was crowded with other athletes who suddenly developed pressing business that required their presence elsewhere. A dozen U.S. athletes chose not to compete and thereby avoided possible disqualification. At the time, it seemed that the tide had turned in favor of the drug testers, but it proved to be just one battle in an ongoing war.

DECIDING WHAT TO TEST

Why use urine? Many athletes object to the loss of privacy involved in having a stranger closely observe the process of urination. Urine is the testing fluid of choice because the metabolites (by-products) of most drugs can be detected in urine. They can also be detected in blood, hair, and saliva.

Although some athletes would prefer to give a blood sample, puncturing the protective barrier of the skin and tapping into the blood supply channels of the body is what is termed an "invasive" procedure, meaning that it opens a potential avenue of infection. Medical ethics discourage unnecessary invasive procedures. A blood test may be on the horizon to detect the presence of the drug erythropoietin and human growth hormone, however. From a legal standpoint, taking blood samples for testing is viewed quite differently from taking urine samples. Consequently, the potential for legal challenges is increased.

What about hair? Drug metabolites do accumulate in hair and tests can reliably demonstrate that a person has used some banned drugs. But hair samples have no timeline, so the drug use may have occurred much earlier. Saliva is still considered an unreliable testing fluid. "There has been some promising work on saliva and sweat and some using hair samples," according to Dr. Baenziger. However, it will be some time before they can be used in sports drug testing, if ever.

Meanwhile, urine is readily available, easily collected, and contains the substances or the metabolites of substances that were taken into the body. The process that leads to obtaining a urine specimen has remained the same over the years. At the Olympic Games, an athlete designated for drug testing is met at the conclusion of the event by an escort who notifies him or her to report to Doping Control. The athlete has one hour after official notification to report, but is accompanied wherever he goes by the escort until he reaches the Doping Control station at the venue. If an athlete wants to drink a beverage in this period, it is supposed to come from a sealed bottle selected by the athlete or his coach from a container of identical sealed bottles.

Once inside the Doping Control station at the venue, the athlete provides a urine specimen under observation by a member of the collection team. This specimen is divided between two vials marked A and B and then sealed in the presence of the athlete. These specially prepared vials have tops that are difficult to remove, even when they are not sealed. Next the vials are packed in special holders and marked with a number. Names of the individual athletes are never marked on the samples that go to the laboratory. For Olympic Games competition, a master list that correlates the names and numbers is kept by Prince De Merode, head of the IOC Medical Commission. After the vials are sealed, a member of the collection team is charged with their custody until they are delivered to the laboratory.

Inside the laboratory, all B samples are refrigerated unopened. Only the A samples are tested initially. When a test is positive, the IOC Medical Commission is notified, and Prince De Merode retrieves the list from his safe and matches the number with a name. The appropriate sports governing body is notified, and it notifies the athlete. Then the B sample is tested. The athlete and/or his representative has the right to be present at the laboratory for the second test. If an athlete declines to come or send a representative, an outsider is recruited to observe the process on his behalf. If the B sample also is positive, the test is reported as positive, and the athlete becomes subject to sanctions by the sports governing body and/or the Olympic Committee of his country.

HOW DRUG TESTING WORKS

Like all substances taken into the body, anabolic steroids are broken down and altered by the process of metabolism. The changes that occur may mean that the parent or original drugs that were taken may not be found in their original form. Therefore, a drug tester also looks for by-products of steroids called metabolites. The distinctive patterns that are formed in these metabolites are like fingerprints in that they are unique and can be matched with the known metabolic "signature" pattern. Each IOC-accredited laboratory maintains an extensive library of these metabolite patterns.

The number of available steroid preparations is large, and the chemical makeup of steroid preparations varies from country to country. Some drugs available in other countries are not used in the United States. In 1992, the androgenic-anabolic steroids category on the IOC banned substances list was renamed anabolic agents to include drugs with purported anabolic (tissue-building) effects. An example of these drugs are the so-called β_2 agonists, which include the drug clenbuterol. Clenbuterol was found in a number of urine samples at the Olympic Games in Barcelona in 1992.

Even though all anabolic steroids have roots in the male sex hormone testosterone, they may be constructed differently. When synthetic compounds are developed, different chemical substitution processes are used to increase the anabolic or tissue-building activity and decrease the androgenic or masculinizing component. In addition, there may be different ester derivatives, particularly nortestosterone and testosterone. (An ester is a compound formed from an alcohol and an acid.)

In very simple terms, developing synthetic compounds is like making a cake. Recipes and ingredients may vary but the final product is always cake. Drug testers have the task of determining exactly what kind of "cake" was consumed from the patterns left by the metabolic residue. Therefore, all of the IOC-approved drug testing laboratories are expected to be able to catch all of the chemical substitutions and alterations. It is a very sophisticated testing system, and a far cry from the first anabolic steroid testing.

The first tests were based on the same principle as many of the current tests for cancer. A radioactive tracer was attached to a specific steroid so it could be tracked to see whether there was an antibody response. This type of test is called a radioimmunoassay (RIA). According to Dr. Craig Kammerer, a senior scientist for Arimenterics, Inc. who was associate director of the UCLA lab in 1984, RIAs were never commercially available because they were not specific enough to use for widespread drug testing, particularly against a body of sophisticated drug users.

Prior to 1984, RIAs (antibody tests) were used for the two different groups of steroids. The agents used were not sensitive for some steroids, however, because they responded to the parent drug rather than to the metabolite. Thus, these tests were neither sufficiently sensitive nor specific to withstand challenge. It is not enough to be "in the ballpark" with drug testing; the method must be very reliable and give the same results each time.

The only currently accepted method of analysis for confirmation and proof of a positive doping test is gas chromatography-mass spectrometry (GC/MS). An extract of the collected urine sample is placed in a gas chromatograph where it gets separated into its

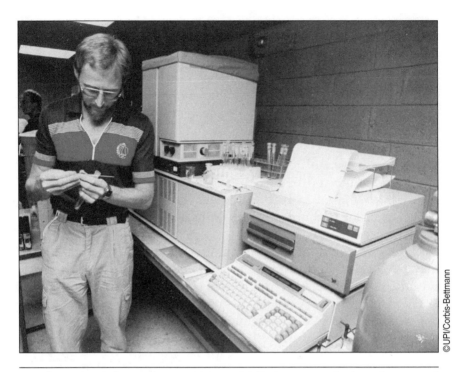

Gas chromatography-mass spectrometry (GC/MS) is currently the only accepted method of analysis for proof of a positive doping test.

component parts. The time that a substance takes to pass through a glass column under a specified set of conditions is one key to its identity. After the sample passes through the gas chromatograph, it goes into a mass spectrometer where its molecules are bombarded with a beam of electrons that fragments them into a distinctive group of pieces or "fingerprints" that are unique for that substance.

The T/E Ratio

When the drug substance being detected is testosterone, the problems of a positive test are compounded by the fact that this substance is produced naturally in the bodies of both men and women. Thus, the presence of testosterone in and of itself is not proof of drug use. The question becomes: How much is too much?

At present, drug testers make that decision by looking at the ratio of testosterone to epitestosterone, another naturally occurring hormone (T/E ratio). Under ordinary conditions, normal adult men

RUNNING INTO TROUBLE

Mary Decker Slaney, considered by many the finest female middle-distance runner in United States history, first competed in the Olympic Games in 1984, where a fall probably cost her a gold medal. Now 38 years old, Slaney is still running—but a question has been raised about how she is maintaining her skill level.

The case has gone on since June 1996, when Slaney had a positive drug test for testosterone at the track and field Olympic Trials. However, because of jurisdictional and procedural differences in the doping rules, she was allowed to compete in her third Olympic Games after she made the team in the 5000-meter event. (She did not advance to the finals at the Games, a fact she attributed to undiagnosed asthma.)

On September 16, 1997, USA Track & Field lifted its suspension and cleared Slaney of doping charges after she and her legal team presented their case to a doping hearing board of the national sports governing body. The panel concluded that she had committed no doping violation. Her attorney attacked the testosterone/epitestosterone ratio test, saying that it is not applicable to women because it can be widely skewed by menstruation or alcohol consumption. While endocrinologists and drug testing experts disagree about how much fluctuation there could be in female T/E ratios, few would agree that it is "widely skewed."

Another female track and field athlete, 400-meter hurdler Sandra Farmer-Patrick, lost her drug hearing before USA Track & Field and has been banned from competition for four years for using testosterone. She also was allowed to compete in Atlanta because her case had not been concluded. The Mary Decker Slaney case may give her grounds for a rehearing.

The international governing body for track and field, IAAF, criticized USA Track & Field for its slow handling of the cases, saying that they should not drag on for months. An IAAF spokesperson said that if the doping commission believes that USA Track & Field was correct in exonerating Slaney, there is no further action to take.

have an average T/E ratio of about 1/1. To avoid penalizing athletes who might naturally produce more testosterone than epitestosterone, however, the IOC set the ratio at 6/1. This ratio has been a cause of great controversy for almost 15 years, with some experts arguing that this test has not been sufficiently validated. This controversy may be the reason that a number of positive T/E ratios have been overturned, invalidated, or not pursued by the responsible sport-governing body.

The T/E ratio of 6 to 1 also has led to one of the greatest abuses of the system. There is a lot of room for steroid use before the laboratories will report the T/E ratio as positive. Even a modest amount of testosterone can be very useful to the athlete, especially women. Moreover, even with a no-notice testing program, an elite athlete may be able to evade detection by using low doses of slow-release testosterone esters or testosterone skin patches (testosterone is delivered through the skin through adhesive patches) or testosterone gels on a continuous basis. Some athletes use private laboratories and monitor their testosterone levels so that the testing limit of 6/1 is not exceeded.

As Dr. Baenziger notes, "One of the things that changed is that a lot of people stopped doing large volumes of drugs. They are doing lower amounts during the training period so they can do harder training and for injury repair." Dr. Catlin says that one immediate action a sports governing body could take is to monitor the results of the T/E ratio over time. Because this ratio is very stable in non-users, he argues, a rise to 5 or 6 would signal drug use, and the governing body could then look into the matter and take whatever action it deemed appropriate.

"We're worried about the athlete who titrates (does his own analysis) and stays at about the level of 4," says Dr. Catlin. "We don't know how much of that there is, but there are some fairly serious cases. In order to link the results from one test to the next, someone in the sports agency has to have the codes and do the linking." (As noted earlier, urine samples are simply coded, and the lab doesn't know the names of the athletes.) He notes that some people in sports administration think that monitoring the T/E ratio is too invasive and too close to privacy issues but adds, "If you want to get rid of the problem, you have do something."

The good news is that Dr. Catlin has developed an alternate test that does not rely on hormone ratios. Instead, this new test involves a direct measure of the carbon isotopes in the urine sample. Because the carbon isotope ratio of pharmaceutical, or synthetic, testosterone is lower than that of testosterone produced within the body, drug testers will be able to see the difference.

Two independent testers have confirmed the accuracy of the test, but it will take time for it to be adopted as the standard test. If this test

THE COST OF DRUG TESTING

Some individuals would like to see drug testing in sports carried out on a bigger scale than has been done previously. A few high schools have even adopted programs to test for steroids. Drug testing is not a cheap system, however, and this cost may be a limiting factor that cannot be overcome.

A number of factors drive the high cost of drug testing. First, the staff must be highly trained to do meticulous laboratory work. For example, the new high-resolution machines that were used at the Atlanta Olympic Games require a fairly extensive training period in order for technicians to be able to operate them effectively. In addition, the testing process calls for the use of expensive reagents.

Steroid testing is more expensive than other types of drug tests. At the beginning of sports drug testing, each test cost approximately $150, a figure that now has dropped to about $120 per test as the number of tests has gone up. However, the cost of testing is particularly pertinent to junior high and high school athletics. The cost of testing hundreds of thousands of high school athletes nationally several times a year would be prohibitively expensive, especially to school systems that have already been forced to cut their funds for athletics because of budget shortfalls.

can tell the difference between natural testosterone and synthetic testosterone, it will halt the wrangling about "naturally high" T/E ratios in athletes with positive tests. Also, some women who have tested positive for high testosterone levels have claimed that the natural production of this hormone varies much more in women than in men and that it can be affected by the monthly hormonal cycles. Dr. Catlin has said that there is no reason to believe that this test will work differently on men and women.

BEATING THE SYSTEM

If drug testing can find such minute amounts of drugs, then why is there a problem? Several problems impact drug testing. Foremost is the fact that steroids are used as training aids, not as a last-minute picker-upper before going out to compete. No drug test can find what is not there. Frequently steroid users can test clean if they know when the test is scheduled; they simply stop taking the drug long enough before the test for the steroid to clear their systems. Some steroids take months to clear, but others may take less than 36 hours.

Moreover, many high school students who use steroids for sports take them mainly in the summer months when they are building up for the fall football or wrestling seasons. Thus, testing at the start of the season will have little or no impact in this group. An announced once-a-year drug test of high school students is simply a waste of money or an exercise in public relations. Only a careless or foolish steroid user will be caught by that type of test.

One method that has been suggested to get around the problem is to do random, unannounced drug tests in the summer. If this proposed change is instituted, the overall success of drug testing could go up. Some might question the cost of such a gain, however. In addition to the simple logistics and expense of testing large numbers of student athletes, some consider this type of drug testing an unwarranted intrusion on privacy. Images of drug testers knocking on the doors of athlete's homes in the middle of the night and demanding urine samples are troubling to many and raise further concerns about the right to privacy.

Yet another area of concern with drug testing relates to how the process is carried out. When all parts of the protocol are executed by the book, the process is fair. However, there are several points in the process when sabotage is at least theoretically possible, beginning with the act of urinating. The reason for the requirement that the athlete be observed while urinating is because there have been instances where individuals used clean urine samples provided by others, even going so far as to inject the urine into their own bladders.

Athletes faced with positive drug tests very often claim that a mistake was made. It is very unlikely in the United States that a substance would be misidentified in either of the IOC-accredited laboratories. The entire process of laboratory testing is not open to the public, however, and thus claims of laboratory error will always find a sympathetic ear in some quarters.

Sometimes athletes say that something they drank or ate after their race was spiked. In the Jessica Foschi case (discussed in chapter 11), that may have happened. At the Olympic Games, athletes are warned not to drink beverages from unsealed containers, and workers are instructed not to hand an athlete even a sealed bottled beverage. The athlete is supposed to make the selection himself from an available cooler.

Dr. Catlin is very aware of the need for meticulous care and watchfulness in carrying out every phase of the drug testing procedure. Noting the importance of the chain of custody, he commented that he could not justify testing samples that might have come from anywhere. He and all the heads of drug laboratory know that unless it can be demonstrated that the urine sample was properly managed from the time the athlete sealed the vials until it reached the laboratory doors, there will be room for doubt.

We have already discussed how athletes sometimes beat the system by staying under the 6/1 T/E ratio. Both Dr. Catlin and Dr. Baenziger also are extremely concerned about the use of agents for which there is, as yet, no drug test. Erythropoietin (EPO), a synthetic agent that stimulates the body to make more oxygen-carrying red blood cells, has replaced blood doping and appears to be gaining ground as a training drug. There is good evidence that increasing the oxygen-releasing capability does have a strong effect on performance, and many athletes have already "field tested" EPO on their own. The danger with this drug is that a miscalculation could lead to a stroke or death. Yet another drug for which no test exists is human growth hormone (hGH), used primarily for its anabolic effects and very popular among athletes who use performance-enhancing drugs. Like EPO, hGH can be used with impunity by athletes, who have no fear of being caught.

New performance-enhancing drugs are appearing on a regular basis in an attempt to defeat the testing process. There were several positive tests for the so-called stimulant bromantan at the Olympic Games in Atlanta. This drug was developed in Russia, and it is reputed to protect the body in a hot environment like Atlanta. Although bromantan did not appear by name on the IOC-banned list until several weeks prior to the Olympics, drug testing officials contended that it was still covered by the "and other related compounds" stipulation. The International Court of Arbitration for Sport overturned the positive tests, saying that athletes were not given sufficient notice that the drug was banned and that the IOC did not sufficiently prove the drug conveyed a competitive advantage.

Dr. Catlin agreed that research continues to develop tests for some newer doping agents, and he said many problems are within the realm of scientific achievement. It is frustrating to those in drug testing to see avenues to increase the effectiveness of drug testing that cannot be taken because of lack of funds. Dr. Catlin contends that it will not be long before a test will be available for EPO, although it may require that athletes also give a blood sample as part of the testing. If technological advances in laboratory techniques now on the horizon make testing itself a different procedure, then there may be a period when sports competition is relatively fair. If the past helps predict the future, however, it may be that while advances in testing are taking place, there also will be other technological breakthroughs that will serve those bent on using drugs.

CHAPTER 6

EDUCATION AND PREVENTION

Education has been a major component of all attempts to control or eliminate illicit drug use. In addition to the several nationwide organizations that are working to decrease recreational drug use, many school districts now mandate steroid education as part of the curriculum covering drugs. Most colleges and sports organizations have formal drug education programs.

The very proliferation of drug education programs sometimes makes it difficult to assess effectiveness. A think tank in Washington, D.C. issued a comprehensive study in 1996 called *Making the Grade: A Guide to School Drug Prevention Programs* to serve as a bridge between the technical research on drug prevention and the hands-on work with youth. Anabolic steroids were not included as a separate item in this guide, however.

At present, education about anabolic steroids is usually added to the general curriculum in many, if not most, school district programs. Most conventional programs stress the very real dangers of recreational drugs, but these dangers don't always correlate with steroids because a user may look better, perform better, and feel healthier! The trouble is that the potential user groups are often not the same. Young people who use alcohol, cocaine, heroin, crack, speed, or other mind-altering chemicals correctly perceive their behavior as risky and likely to draw public disapproval (at the least) or trouble with the law. They may be rebelling, self-medicating, or succumbing to peer pressure in their use. On the other hand, a sizable portion of young athletes who take steroids wouldn't dream of using recreational drugs. They don't drink, don't smoke, are careful about diet, and generally fit the mainstream ideal.

Even among steroid users who do use other illicit drugs, the vast majority do not use steroids to alter their mood or escape reality, as is the case with the recreational drugs they use. Steroid-using athletes, especially those at the elite level, argue that not only are they not

PAT CONNOLLY

Pat Connolly is a woman who knows what it's like both to compete and coach at the top. A former Olympian, Connolly was the coach of the great Olympic champion sprinter Evelyn Ashford. Her keen interest in preventing steroid use comes from watching steroid users firsthand. She has worked with a number of official sports committees seeking to keep steroids out of sports. "Women have only begun to explore their potential physically," she says. "To short-circuit that with drugs is a great disservice because then a woman never knows how good she could be."

She tells young women that when a coach, trainer, or other supporting person whispers to them that they could be much better if they used steroids not to listen because they are being undermined psychologically. "When coaches push performance drugs, they are telling the athlete they don't believe in her, that she isn't good enough as she is," Connolly says, adding that young women who take the drug route may never know what they could have been on their own. "You have to find out how good you are, not how good your pharmacist is," she insists.

Ashford is, in Connolly's mind, "the greatest sprinter ever to run down the track," even if her records have been eclipsed by women rumored to take performance-enhancing drugs. Ashford herself has been quoted as saying she would run until her legs fell off because she loved the feel of running. "It wasn't about the gold medal; it was about the performance," says Connolly, adding that the best women athletes compete for the joy of the sport and that steroid use takes away the pleasure of accomplishment.

trying to avoid reality, they are confronting it! These athletes contend that they use steroids to maintain parity with other drug-using athletes or to survive in a society that increasingly embraces "win-at-all-costs" and "it's-only-cheating-if-you-get-caught" philosophies. The only real philosophical intersection between steroid use and other drug use is a belief in the value of pharmaceuticals, that pills or injections can provide solutions.

The implication here for educational efforts is that the two kinds of drug use perhaps should not be addressed together, as is the case now with many established programs. If the educational effort is not well-founded, it runs the risk of whetting youthful interest in taking steroids. When that curiosity is roused, today's youth don't have to start hanging out at the gym or take up bodybuilding. Information is no further away than the Internet. A recent casual survey that made use of only one of the many search engines available on the Internet found approximately 5,000 steroid references! Many contained anti-steroid messages, but many more did not. The age of the computer makes it much easier for word to spread about new drugs and sources of supply.

The current situation may seem to be a depressing no-win position for those of us who do see the very real dangers in steroid use. We have known for decades that athletes can achieve meaningful muscle and strength gains on their own with proper strength training and diet, without steroids. When they make these gains through their own efforts, the healthful effects last a lifetime, and the athletes gain additional confidence in their abilities.

Experts on drugs and sports agree that a national prevention effort is badly needed. One fact that has emerged is that successful intervention is early intervention. Because 4 percent or more of high school boys and more than 2 percent or more of junior high school boys have tried steroids, it is quite reasonable to initiate educational efforts at the junior high and middle school levels.

Drug testing was always intended to be paired with educational programs. It just has taken more time to develop the educational model. Most early attempts at interventions, although undoubtedly well-intentioned, consisted of a one-time appeal such as showing a video, placing a poster in the locker room, or having an expert give a lecture. These limited strategies were often formulated quickly and based in large part on strategies that have been used against street drugs, albeit with questionable efficacy there also. To their surprise and dismay, educators and coaches soon found that this type of intervention seemed only to enhance interest in steroids, even when athletes were told that steroids and other performance-enhancing drugs have potentially serious harmful effects on health and that they unfairly influence the outcome of competition.

Now that many athletes have experienced firsthand the disadvantages of competing against steroid-using athletes and how these drugs subvert ethical and sportsmanlike standards, they may be a more receptive audience. Enough publicity has been given to bad physical, mental, and legal outcomes in steroid users that most young athletes know they have a definite downside. Conversations with Olympic and other elite athletes have convinced us that there is growing support against performance-enhancing drugs. The time may be ripe for an all-out prevention effort because there is finally some good news about prevention.

THE SEARCH FOR AN EDUCATIONAL MODEL

Prevention of steroid use has been a major theme of the work of Linn Goldberg, MD, and others at the Human Performance Laboratory at the Oregon Health Sciences University, Portland, Oregon. After more than 10 years of study on the best ways to reach potential users while they are still adolescents, they now believe they know what works and what doesn't. "Scare tactics head the list of unsuccessful ways to prevent steroid use," Dr. Goldberg, a professor of medicine at the university, says emphatically. "Nor can you expect success with a perfunctory lecture at the start of the sports season. The program we developed that appears to have the most effect is global. It affects behavioral intent, attitudes toward drug use, body image, and mediators that can stimulate drug use. It involves the coach, the family, and the team, not just the athlete. Talking to the individual is not enough. We have to affect the whole social sphere of influence."

Most coaches already understand very well the motivation that can be applied through the social sphere of influence, and successful ones use that technique to achieve their sports-related and personal goals. When the social sphere of influence becomes negative, the results are just as striking. There have been several instances (the universities of Oklahoma, Miami, and Nebraska come to mind) where collegiate football programs have been as well-known for off-the-field problems, including arrests, as their on-the-field successes. The social sphere of influence is a powerful tool.

When the Oregon researchers first began looking at ways to influence high school football players in their state, their first step was to identify effective methods of getting their message across. Football players in the study were divided into three groups. The first group listened to medical students present a lecture and viewed slides that gave a balanced presentation about the risks and potential benefits of steroids. A second group also heard a lecture given by a medical student, but only the negative aspects of steroid use were presented. The third group received a written handout on steroids. Which intervention gave the best results? Interest in using steroids was unchanged or increased in all three groups! Dr. Goldberg explains that this result occurred because educational strategies that rely only on factual information frequently fail to alter behavior. People need more than just facts; they need motivation. Undaunted, the researchers pressed on.

The ATLAS Prevention Program

Now, after five years of development and five more years of refining the pilot program, the Adolescents Training and Learning to Avoid Steroids (ATLAS) Prevention Program was born (see figure 6.1). A formal evaluation of ATLAS showed that participants, relative to a control group, were less interested in trying steroids, had a better understanding of the positive and negative effects of steroids, had better drug refusal skills, and had improved nutrition and eating habits.

The ATLAS program involves 14 sessions with three main information modules:

■ Weight training skills
■ Nutritional information for sports
■ Anabolic steroids education

The education module includes everything that the Oregon researchers have learned about using the social sphere approach. This approach involves providing and demonstrating practical information on alternatives to steroid use and presenting other information in an

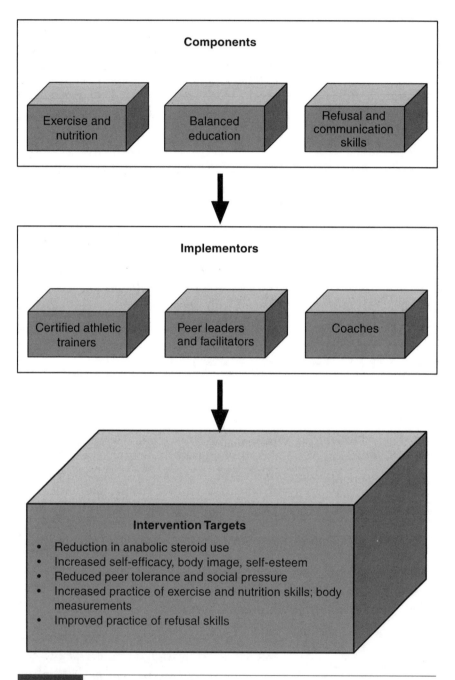

Components

Exercise and nutrition

Balanced education

Refusal and communication skills

Implementors

Certified athletic trainers

Peer leaders and facilitators

Coaches

Intervention Targets

- Reduction in anabolic steroid use
- Increased self-efficacy, body image, self-esteem
- Reduced peer tolerance and social pressure
- Increased practice of exercise and nutrition skills; body measurements
- Improved practice of refusal skills

FIGURE 6.1   The ATLAS Program is a way to educate young people about alternatives to steroids.

Data courtesy of Dr. Linn Goldberg.

effective format. "We think it's important to give kids a reasonable alternative to drug use for their athletic enhancement," says Dr. Goldberg. "One is to teach weight training skills. Many adolescent kids don't have these skills and are not taught by coaches who have the skills themselves."

Scientific weight training is a development of relatively modern times and the concepts of circuit training and progressive development are not as widely known as they deserve to be. Too often, weight training is a poorly supervised activity that does little if anything to add to an athlete's physical development. In the Oregon program, however, 7 of the 14 sessions are conducted in the weight room.

Dr. Goldberg says that adolescence is a great time to begin weight training. "If a teenage boy didn't do anything but sit on a couch, his strength would increase four-fold as his natural hormonal development moves him toward adult strength," Dr. Goldberg observed, adding that his program takes advantage of those normal physiological changes. The universal adolescent concern for appearance is a major reason cited by teenagers who take steroids. By using effective non-drug methods of physical training, teenagers can improve their body image and increase self-esteem.

The second important area where the available scientific knowledge doesn't always reach the athlete is sports nutrition. Just as a team may have competition goals and weight training goals, it also should have nutrition goals. Gains in muscle strength and size that are generated by weight training appear to be enhanced by protein intake that exceeds the recommended daily allowance. "Don't just tell them about nutrition," cautions Dr. Goldberg, who notes that although nutrition is a standard unit for high school health classes, sports nutrition is not.

Athletes need to understand that dietary fuels for competition and muscle development differ from those needed for ordinary activity. His volunteer instructors go through a program that provides students with information on relevant topics, such as how to order food in a restaurant to get high-octane energy or what they should eat before or after a workout. When athletes start eating a proper sports nutrition diet, most see positive changes in athletic performance. "Proper diet" does not mean loading up with vitamins, dietary supplements, or amino acids, many of which are promptly washed out of the body in urine. The emphasis is on a healthy diet that can be devised by proper meal planning. Too few athletes know how to do that.

The third arm of the program is instruction about anabolic steroids. This information is given in a balanced presentation that does not focus only on negatives because the Oregon group learned early in their pilot study research that accentuating the negative turned kids off. The high school football players who heard only about unwanted side effects like breast growth, hair loss, or cholesterol elevation were essentially unmoved in their beliefs about steroids when they were tested later about changes in their attitudes. Dr. Goldberg theorizes that a lack of any acknowledgment of possible steroid benefit may have appeared to be too biased to be credible. Armed with that knowledge, the steroid education component gives both the good and bad effects of steroid use.

The Oregon team also teaches prevalence of steroid use. Many athletes think it is more widespread than it is (according to figures from research studies), and they rationalize their own use by saying everybody does it. Although 4 to 11 percent of high school boys state that they have used steroids at one time or another, 89 to 96 percent have not used steroids.

The steroid prevention program is given in training sessions that make use of peer facilitators and discussion groups. Although medical students still serve as training coordinators, they are not "talking heads," or experts who just drop in and give a lecture. Peer facilitators are nominated by other players and receive a day of special training before the program begins. The unique position of the peer leader as a role model for his teammates is stressed. Upperclassmen pair up with younger players in a "buddy system," wherein older players help reinforce the lessons.

Sessions include various learning exercises that have been devised to stimulate players to look critically at claims made for steroids. For instance, when they examine magazines that glorify bodybuilding, they also see and discuss the advertising in the magazine for hair replacements or breast reductions so that they understand that acceleration of male pattern balding and breast development are negative outcomes of steroid use. This approach helps student athletes to see the fine print beyond the big claims. Athletes also learn refusal skills (how to say no) that are backed by realistic and specific reasons they can use if they are approached about trying steroids.

Four booster sessions are scheduled each year because retraining has been shown to reinforce the initial interventions. The review covers factual information about steroids, nutrition and exercise, and refusal skills. After athletes complete the program, they are tested again about their attitudes toward drug use. Dr. Goldberg and his fellow researchers have found that this fairly labor-intensive program that relies on the combination of knowledge and peer participation and support from the team works to reduce interest in steroids.

ANOTHER VOICE

Nancy Kennedy, DrPH (doctor of public health), is another individual who recognizes the complexity of steroid prevention. In her work at the Center for Substance Abuse Prevention (CSAP) within the Department of Health and Human Services, she has seen enough data to conclude that steroid education must be interwoven with other education and that the individual, peer, family, school, workplace, and community must be supportive of non-steroid using athletes. Speaking at the 1994 meeting of the American Public Health Association, Dr. Kennedy said, "Any prevention program must address these different forces: attitudes, personality, family, social, and environmental."

She noted that the classic method of eliminating a public health problem has been to attack the causative agent. In drug abuse, the agent is often considered to be the drug itself. To an extent, that approach works with drugs like cocaine and marijuana. Steroids cannot be handled in this manner, however, because they still are unrecognized (by the public) as a drug, and this condition hampers prevention efforts. Nor does she think the outlook for prevention of steroids is optimistic. "Not only is there a disinclination to view them as harmful drugs, every time an athlete is found to be a user, it has been in the successful mode. We don't have a negative mode for steroids," she commented.

In Dr. Kennedy's view, athletes who have been publicly linked to steroid use have been seen as successful people. Arnold Schwarzenegger comes to mind. Even when an athlete does have a negative outcome, such as Steve Courson, it usually happens after the athlete's competitive years and is not publicly visible.

Moreover, Dr. Kennedy sees the social environment for steroids as encouraging, in both subtle and not so subtle ways, by embracing a "win at all costs," "appearance is everything" mentality. "To really change behavior, a person must internalize how that behavior is controlling his life," says Dr. Kennedy. That is easier with drugs such as cocaine and heroin because a user generally functions at a low level and frequently looks that way. Steroid users, on the other hand, may function at a high level and look good.

Teens may resist traditional interventions aimed at preventing illicit marijuana or cocaine use because their goals, such as getting high and having unusual experiences, are antagonistic to adult values. On the other hand, steroid abusers may have goals like enhanced appearance and improved athletic performance that are consistent with adult values and thereby escape close scrutiny of their actions. "When you take steroids and look in a mirror," Dr. Kennedy continued, "you probably look good and that makes it difficult to change the drug-taking behavior. If you value looking good and doing well, steroids may help you do that."

She suggests one possible method of effecting change is by appealing to personal integrity. When individuals come to view the use of steroids and other performance-enhancing drugs as a form of cheating, there will be motivation for change, and recent conversations with Olympic athletes convince us that many do see steroid use as cheating. That alone, however, is not enough, says Dr. Kennedy, adding that reinforcement for change must also come from the family, peers, and community of the user. She and the Oregon group find common ground about the best chance for success against steroid abuse in that both believe motivation must come from the social sphere of influence.

The fact that cultural attitudes have a strong influence on public behavior is demonstrated in Mexico where drugs of all varieties are widely available and can be purchased without a prescription. Nevertheless, with the exception of alcohol and tobacco, drug usage rates for Hispanic families are low. "We hypothesize that it has something to do with the fact that Hispanic families are close-knit and that there is a negative value associated with drug use," says Dr. Kennedy. Prevention of steroid use in the United States may well demand that same type of support, in which the community and/or society disapproves strongly of using drugs to enhance athletics. Conversely, so long as the community and/or society accepts drug use as normal, motivation for change will not be high.

Dr. Kennedy said her work at CSAP and earlier as an epidemiologist at the National Institute on Drug Abuse has convinced her of the importance of finding the best point of intervention. With adoles-

JIM KELLY

Jim Kelly, recently retired quarterback of the Buffalo Bills, is an athlete who knows what it takes to succeed at the highest level of football, and he likes to see youngsters get started on the right path. His message to parents is, "Encouragement is very important. Children have an enormous amount of pressure on them today, and therefore, a parent needs to concentrate on positive reinforcement. Parents should press a gifted athlete to make the most of his or her gift, but not so hard that it turns the child off to the very thing God has blessed him with."

Because young athletes are curious about steroids and may be a target for individuals who tell them drugs are the answer, Kelly was asked what advice he might give athletes just beginning careers about performance-enhancing drugs. "Nowadays, all athletes must be clean in every sport," he said. "Therefore it is critical to success as an athlete to start clean and stay clean. Otherwise, your misdeeds will come back to haunt you and ruin your chance to participate at the next level."

Keeping perspective on athletics is important also, and Kelly sums it up by saying, "Winning is definitely the bottom line, but guys who don't concentrate on anything but winning should be avoided. There will always be guys with that attitude, but I think that the level of success they attain will always be hurt by it."

Kelly was regarded as one of the top quarterbacks in the NFL. He believes steroid use is declining in favor of emphasis on technical skills, off-season conditioning, and proper diet. He is certain steroids are no substitute for talent. "If you don't have what it takes to get the job done, no man-made substance is going to get you there," he says. "I think an informed athlete is a successful athlete. If you're not using your head in today's sports scene, then you are definitely out of style."

cents, early intervention is mandatory because teens have already learned that physical appearance is important in this culture. She has found that both teenage boys and girls are interested in obtaining information about anabolic steroids, and their customary sources may not give a balanced picture.

Several studies of high school students have shown that the most popular sources of information for users were friends, people at gyms, television, muscle magazines, health professionals, and newspapers. Television was the most popular information source among

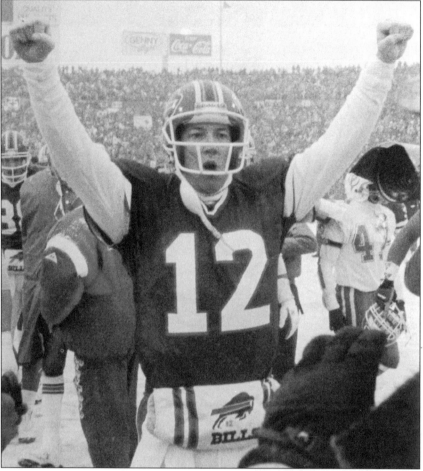

©UPI/Corbis-Bettmann

Former NFL star quarterback Jim Kelly advises young athletes to "start clean and stay clean."

non-users, according to one study. In that group, 11 percent of non-users cited physicians and health professionals as sources of information. Teachers and coaches are not mentioned often as sources of steroid information, which suggests that teachers and coaches might have some impact on prevention if they could serve as an information source in a non-threatening, objective way. Dr. Kennedy says when teens perceive the environment as threatening, they will not ask questions.

Unspoken messages can encourage steroid use, Dr. Kennedy observed, adding that knowing the messages and counterbalancing or eliminating them makes it less likely that steroids will be attractive to athletes. Drug use becomes more attractive when the following messages are present:

- The concept of sports as fun is superseded by sports as a business.
- There is a spirit of winning at all costs.
- There is overemphasis on physical attributes for feelings of self-worth.
- There is a search for shortcuts, for instant gratification versus long-term goals.
- Money and appearance are valued above health.
- Drugs are accepted as a way to solve problems and get quick results.
- There are financial rewards for winning.

Schools and individuals, such as coaches and teachers, can help the prevention effort by setting limits in the form of appropriate drug policies, according to Dr. Kennedy. A school drug policy should prohibit possession, use, or distribution of steroids by athletes or staff. Orientation programs should be held in conditioning facilities like gyms and weight rooms. Regular assessments of body mass, body fat, and strength of athletes are appropriate, she continued, adding that parents should receive reports giving this information. A description of the school's strength training program philosophy and goals for athletic conditioning also should be sent to the parents of all athletes, Dr. Kennedy believes. Athletes and parents may be asked to sign a comprehensive statement against steroid use as a prerequisite to participating in a conditioning program.

A comprehensive prevention program also calls for watching for signs of steroid use and being ready to intervene when they are present. Doctors can help in the anti-steroid effort by using risk screening assessment for their teen patients and by asking about possible steroid use during pre-season physicals or while treating injuries or other illnesses. Strength coaches, trainers, or conditioning supervisors should be especially alert to the signs and symptoms of steroid use, and inform parents when two or more of the following symptoms are apparent:

- Sudden increases in strength, body weight, or lean body mass beyond what would be reasonably expected from normal growth and development and training alone

- Acne or puffiness caused by fluid retention
- Personality changes (hyperactive behavior, aggression, hostility, depression)
- Obsessive commitment to conditioning, strength, or physique as an end in itself
- The presence of drug paraphernalia
- Appearance of needle marks, particularly in large muscle groups such as buttocks and thighs
- Deepening of the voice (women only)
- Masculinization, such as male pattern hair growth on face and body (women only)
- Shrinkage of mammary glands (women only)

Dr. Kennedy is concerned that too many people still believe that drug testing is an effective prevention strategy, adding that this mistaken belief can result in a false sense of security on the part of parents, teachers and coaches. She stresses that there is no substitute for the personal involvement of those around an athlete in preventing drug use. With the information now available on steroid prevention strategies that can be successful, athletes may once again compete on a level playing field if the entire community, athlete, coach, trainer, family, friends, school officials, and fans, participate in the group effort.

CHAPTER 7

STEROIDS AND THE LAW

The legal issues that pertain to steroid use are complicated in that there are several ways users can run afoul of the law or face disciplinary action by a sports governing body. Areas of concern include the following:

- **Sports drug testing.** An athlete who fails a drug test for steroids may be banned from competing in his sport for a period of time, usually two years or more.

- **Steroid trafficking**. The federal government and all state governments have laws against the distribution, possession, or prescription of anabolic steroids for nonmedical use.

- **Crimes committed while taking steroids**. A steroid user whose aggressive feelings are beyond control may face legal action for such crimes as assault and battery, domestic violence, and other misdemeanors and felonies associated with loss of control.

SPORTS DRUG TESTING

Although drug testing has been part of sports for more than 25 years, it still is a source of disagreement between those who see it as an intrusive and unnecessary element and those who credit it with trying to maintain standards of fair competition. An often cited point is that participating in sports is not a right but a privilege, and most of the legal decisions upholding testing are based on that principle. This principle derives from the fact that sports organizations are, by and large, private associations, and such membership is an intangible property right. Traditionally, the courts have given private associations wide latitude to control and define those rights. In theory, drug testing appears to be a sports-specific method to level the playing field by preventing chemically-induced advantages for steroid users.

There are both general and sports-specific reasons why sports governing bodies may desire drug testing. General reasons include protecting the long-term physical and mental health of athletes and identifying "problem" athletes. What is clear is that when private organizations do propose testing athletes for drugs, a criterion of the testing program should be that clear evidence can be demonstrated of a relationship between use of the banned drugs and their adverse effects on performance, health, or quality of the competition.

Those who believe in the concept of drug testing can point to several successful outcomes. For instance, drug testing has eliminated many, but not all, drugs that must be taken at the time of competition to be effective. Examples of these drugs are amphetamines and beta blockers, and finding these chemicals is just a simple day at the office in the drug laboratories.

What drug testing has not eliminated are the so-called training drugs, including anabolic steroids, that are taken to permit athletes to do harder and longer workouts. These drugs confer a significant advantage, and when the drug use is timed right with the competitions, the traces are long gone by the time the urine sample is requested.

Sometimes a miscalculation or a metabolic act of fate does leave the drug user exposed with steroids or their metabolites in his or her body at the time of testing. That was the case with Canadian sprinter Ben Johnson in 1988. As part of the full-scale investigation that followed, the physician who supplied Johnson with the steroid stanozolol became the target of a probe that uncovered an extensive distribution network among elite athletes that included exchanging steroids for cocaine. Several hundred thousand dosage units of steroids were distributed on a monthly basis in Canada, the United States, and some of the Caribbean islands. This network seemed like a well-organized drug-taking program.

Another major drawback of any widespread testing program is the cost. Drug testing at each of the last three Summer Olympic Games exceeded 2 million dollars. If every high school football

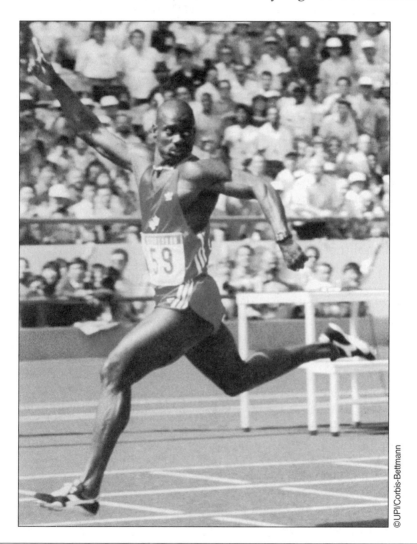

©UPI/Corbis-Bettmann

Johnson's positive steroid test re-ignited the issue of fair play in sports, not to mention the long-term health consequences of steroid use.

player in the United States were tested just once yearly, it would cost more than 100 million dollars. The question is whether scarce resources should be used in this manner.

Athletes' Rights

Putting aside for a moment any discussion of the effectiveness of drug testing, there have always been constitutional issues about whether drug testing is warranted. These issues include the 4th Amendment protection against unreasonable search and seizure, the 14th Amendment due process issues, and the 5th Amendment protection against self-incrimination.

The due process concern is that the procedures must observe a basic principle of fairness. There should be timely notification of a positive test, an opportunity for the singled-out athlete to appear and refute the findings, and an appeals process for correction of any major errors. It is very important to athletes to have an opportunity to explain an adverse finding and/or request another testing for confirmation. Some of the successful challenges to disqualification for positive drug tests have come about because of a lack of due process for the athlete. Examples include an athlete not being given reasonable notice to appear to be tested or not being properly advised of his appeal rights. When attorneys mount a legal challenge to a positive drug test, due process is the area most often attacked.

The privacy issue is cited most often by athletes who resent having an observer watch them urinate. The fact is that although they may believe that they are guaranteed a right to privacy, the Constitution itself does not do that, and the notion that individuals have a right to privacy is a relatively recent legal development. Various state constitutions and state laws do provide specific privacy protection, however, and these laws have been used in several suits brought by athletes, including the most recent case brought by an Oregon school student, James Acton. In that important case, the U.S. Supreme Court upheld the constitutionality of sports drug testing in its June 26, 1995 decision (Vernonia School District 47J versus Acton).

The Acton case was not the first protesting sports drug testing. Almost as soon as collegiate drug testing programs were instituted in 1986, the first legal actions against the NCAA were filed—and lost. The first successful action was filed by a Stanford University diver in November 1987. She maintained that the tests were degrading,

THE ACTON CASE

During the 1992 school year, James Acton was a seventh grade student who wanted to play football. The school district required all members of the team and their parents to sign a consent form for random urinalysis tests. The Actons refused to sign the form and James was suspended from interscholastic athletics. The Actons then brought suit charging that the school policy violated James' right to be free from unreasonable government searches under both the Fourth Amendment and Article 1, Section 9 of the Oregon Constitution.

After the federal district court upheld the constitutionality of the school policy, the Actons appealed. The federal appeals court in San Francisco reversed the lower court decision. In agreeing with the Actons, the appeals court made the type of drug testing James was facing illegal in the nine western states in its jurisdiction. The U.S. Supreme Court upheld the constitutionality of the testing procedure, however. The arguments in favor of a drug testing policy for school students is that it is prompted by serious questions of a safety nature and that a random suspicionless drug testing program does not discriminate against any individual.

Speaking for the Court, Justice Antonin Scalia said that the State could exercise a greater degree of supervision and control over schoolchildren than it could over free adults. The Court also said that in order to participate in sports, the athlete must make some concession to the public interest in conducting athletics in a drug-free setting. It also said that the school drug testing policy was a response to drug usage by athletes.

---

invaded her privacy, and constituted an illegal search. Stanford joined the suit and the courts agreed that it was inappropriate to treat athletes as if they were suspected criminals. Since that time, there have been any number of other legal actions, but the courts have, in general, consistently upheld the right of private organizations, such as the National Collegiate Athletic Association (NCAA), the International Olympic Committee (IOC), or the National Football League (NFL) to conduct drug testing. The 1995 Supreme Court decision in the Acton case lends weight to that position.

A significant aspect of steroid drug testing is that the testing process must be different from other drug testing in order to be effective. For instance, an announced one-time steroid test is a waste of money. The athlete simply stops taking the drug long enough before testing to allow the drug or its by-products to leave his or her body. Random, unannounced tests can be somewhat more effective, but they carry a much greater risk of becoming an intrusion into an athlete's private life. Athletes are very suspicious of such tests because they are concerned about the possibility of sabotage. Suppose a drug tester shows up at a workout one day, taps an athlete on the shoulder, and says, "You, come with me." That athlete has every right to be very concerned about matters such as the fairness of the testing selection process, the chain of custody during transport to the testing laboratory, and due process.

Some observers of drug testing and many athletes are concerned that some sports organizations are inconsistent or uneven in their publication of and sanctions for positive tests. Consequently, these organizations could be vulnerable to lawsuits that allege selective application of standards. In addition, if a sports organization receives notification of positive drug tests but chooses not to impose sanctions or publicize the results, an intriguing question arises about the legal liability of the enforcement organization, the sports governing body. Speculation has been advanced that an organization that knows about a positive test but imposes no sanction assumes the liability for the future adverse health effects that athlete may incur from his drug use. If true, this could have great relevance for the NFL, where there has been a great deal of steroid use among players.

In any event, because an athlete with a positive drug test can be deprived of his right to compete in national and international events, it is extremely important to reach an agreement on how to conduct drug testing of athletes so that the process is fair for all. At this point, there is so much mistrust about drug testing that it will take time before the foundation of agreement can be developed wherein athletes feel their legal rights are protected and sports organizations feel they are safeguarding the integrity of the competition.

STEROIDS AS A CONTROLLED SUBSTANCE

Anabolic steroids became a Schedule III controlled substance when President George Bush signed the Anabolic Steroid Control Act of

1990 on November 28 of that year. Congress enacted this act in response to increased public recognition of steroids as dangerous drugs and because of revelations about the extent of steroid use in sports, especially among adolescents, as well as in occupations requiring strength and power, such as law enforcement. In addition to underscoring the seriousness of the problem, the act enhanced the ability of law enforcement agencies to address the problem.

Numerous state and federal laws relating to steroids also were enacted during the late 1980s and early 1990s, and a federal interagency task force was formed in 1990 to provide a coordinated federal approach to this public health problem, including interrupting the business lines of black market steroid dealers and distributors. Since then, the courts have become increasingly involved in dealing with suppliers. Most cases deal with the distribution of large amounts of drugs.

In Detroit, more than 2 million dosage units of legitimate and counterfeit steroids were seized by federal agents as part of a haul that also included cocaine, marijuana, and prescription drugs. In all, 46 arrests were made, including four on homicide charges. In Boston, a former Mr. Universe pleaded guilty to a 14-count indictment that charged him with being the East Coast distributor for an international trafficker in steroids. Deliveries and seizures totaled in excess of 260,000 dosage units. He was sentenced to four months in prison. A Miami investigation turned up a gym owner who was identified as the source of supply of anabolic steroids for a ring. More than 100,000 dosage units were seized. The trafficker was sentenced to eight years in prison and fined 5,000 dollars.

These are just a few examples of the 355 anabolic steroid investigations that were initiated by the Drug Enforcement Administration (DEA) between February 1991 and February 1995. There have been more than 400 arrests, and more than 200 defendants have been convicted. Because of the way criminal penalties were set up for steroid infractions, however, an individual brought to court on charges of distribution or selling steroids must be a national level dealer to get more than a slap on the wrist and/or a short visit to a "country club" prison. For this reason, enforcement agents often do not bother pursuing small cases because the costs of prosecution vastly outweigh any penalties that will be assessed.

Moreover, even though the legal apparatus to control steroid trafficking is there, enforcement agents already are struggling to handle the problems of importation, distribution, sales, and use of such drugs as cocaine and heroin. Based on what we know about the physical, psychological, or social effects of steroids, it is neither realistic nor appropriate that enforcement efforts for steroids should take precedent over those for more harmful drugs. On the other hand, this line of reasoning should not be used as a rationale for a lack of effective action against steroids.

Nevertheless, the prospect that limited government resources can be stretched to cover yet another class of drugs is not optimistic, especially now that recreational drug use appears to be on an upswing. The availability of anabolic steroids in this country suggests there is some reason to believe that the United States may simply not have the police manpower effectively to deal with catching and punishing sellers of anabolic steroids and other performance-enhancing drugs.

In the early days of steroids, most athletes obtained them by prescription from a doctor or from another athlete. A black market grew to meet the demand, and veterinary steroids also came into use. Even though anabolic steroids are now a controlled substance, doctors may still prescribe steroids under certain circumstances, but records of prescriptions are kept and sales are regulated.

Although the Anabolic Steroid Control Act undoubtedly has deterred most health professionals from prescribing steroids for non-medical use, an estimated 10 percent of illicit users still obtain their drugs from a physician, pharmacist, or veterinarian. Most U.S. steroid users now deal with black market sources when they want to make a buy. Many of these sources also deal in other illicit drugs such as cocaine and marijuana. There have been instances of high school kids selling steroids out of their lockers, but the primary supply source is found in weight training gyms and, to a lesser extent, mail order sources. The Internet also serves as a source for drug information and sales outlets.

Like all other illegal drugs, anabolic steroids are a big business. The black market in steroids and other sports drugs is estimated to be more than 400 million dollars in annual retail sales. As steroid use has become increasingly criminalized, the distribution network has shifted from the illegal diversion of steroids legally manufactured in the United States to a distribution network fed by steroids smuggled in from foreign countries. European and South American countries seem to be the primary source area for steroids coming into the United States. Steroids produced in eastern Europe are frequently sent through bases in western Europe en route to the United States. Some of these foreign clandestine laboratories put out substandard or potentially dangerous products or, conversely, products that claim to be steroids but which contain no active substances.

In Mexico, anabolic steroids (and almost all other drugs that require a doctor's prescription in the United States) can be purchased over the counter. Many users simply cross the border, purchase steroids, and attempt to smuggle them into this country. Because Russian and other European steroids are generally viewed (erroneously) as more effective than Mexican steroids, they are more attractive to black market purchasers. One particularly dishonest dealer who knew this fact had labels made up to indicate an East German source of supply when, in fact, the steroids were made in a secret U.S. laboratory.

Anabolic steroids intended for animals often end up being taken by humans. Steroids are legitimate treatment for animals, especially horses and dogs, and some veterinarians have become both a direct and indirect source for individuals seeking steroids for their own use. The use of steroids for horses is a practice that has caused considerable controversy in the racing world, particularly now that more is known about the effects of the drugs. In addition, some horsemen feel it unfairly affects the nature of horse racing. Veterinary sources are sometimes used to obtain the diuretic Lasix, which is used by some wrestlers and other athletes who need to "make weight." This drug is often given to horses, and it carries a health risk to humans who use it for sports purposes.

Legalization as an Option

One suggestion that has been the subject of heated debate is to legalize the use of steroids, both in society and in sport. Some have called this posture "accepting reality" and say that it would lessen the level of hypocrisy in sports. It would also eliminate the law enforcement costs associated with steroid use. An Australian physician has suggested that the drugs should be legalized, and doctors should monitor athletes who take them. In an article in an Australian medical journal, he observed that danger is not a deterrent to use, citing alcohol and hard drugs as examples. In his opinion, doctors should operate from a position of trying to reduce the harm caused by steroids.

Two levels of authority would be involved if such a legalization were to take place. First, federal and state laws regarding the importation, possession, distribution, and prescription of anabolic steroids would have to be changed. Second, the bans on steroids now in place for virtually every sport would have to be rescinded.

Legalization of steroids in sport might lessen hypocrisy, but it would place an extremely heavy burden on individual athletes who then would be forced either to take drugs known to be harmful or compete at a disadvantage. Although drug testing has more than a few frailties, it has essentially eliminated the use of some dangerous drugs, such as amphetamines, and significantly decreased the dosages of others, as is the case with anabolic steroids.

Therefore, if we did legalize drugs in sport, that would mark the end of any traditional ideals of sport and competition. For that reason alone, legalization of steroids is not acceptable at this time.

Conference on Steroid Abuse

The first International Conference on Abuse and Trafficking of Anabolic Steroids was held in 1993 in Prague, Czech Republic. The conference was the first of its kind in having a broader context than just steroids use by athletes. It was intended to develop recognition of the consequences of steroid abuse, to examine steroid trafficking at the national and international levels, and to explore appropriate responses to the problem of steroid abuse. In addition to the individual representatives from 19 countries, the International Criminal Police Organization (ICPO)/Interpol, the IOC, the International Narcotics Control Board, the World Health Organization, the U.S. Department of State, the U.S. Food and Drug Administration, and the U.S. Drug Enforcement Administration also sent representatives.

Delegates were told that the evidence of adverse physical and psychological effects is growing, including an increase in the amount of steroid-associated aggression and the development of dependency on steroids. Dr. Michael S. Bahrke, discussed the nature of anabolic steroid abuse, noting that many steroid users are not heavily involved in sports, although they usually are doing intensive weight training. Few in this group of users have ever undergone urine testing for steroid detection. The occupations of some of the individuals in a steroid research project Dr. Bahrke directed in Chicago included personal fitness trainers, night club bouncers, gym owners/ managers, firefighters, and kickboxers.

One finding of the Prague conference was the urgent need for increased health, psychological, and epidemiological research and dissemination of scientific knowledge to authorities. Many health professionals do not have current information about anabolic steroid use. Steroid research funding is not expected to improve during the present budget-cutting period, however.

Nevertheless, researchers have a reason to step up research because steroids often are being used in ways (such as high doses and multiple steroids taken simultaneously in combination with other illicit drugs) that are different from any type of medical therapy; as a result, the potential side effects are difficult to anticipate. Also, the populations using steroids include large numbers of teens and young adults who are still in the last phases of growth and development, a process that, theoretically, could be disrupted seriously by taking steroids. Although the short-term harmful effects of steroid use have been documented, the long-term effects are still unknown, and only research can provide those answers.

STEROID CRIME

Taken over time and in high doses, steroids may possibly bring about significant adverse personality changes in some users. Dr. Precilla Choi, a former power lifter who is a lecturer in health psychology at the University of Nottingham in the United Kingdom, argues that because the clinical literature does state that therapeutic doses of steroids (doses that are given as medical therapy) reduce fatigue and produce increased aggression, euphoria, and changes in sex drive and mood, it is reasonable to assume that massive doses of steroids (the amounts taken by some users) would also produce psychological effects.

Fights in bars, insults traded at the gym, domestic violence, sudden irrational acts, and angry blow-ups are common manifestations of the sometimes explosive personality changes that have been observed. A Chicago radio personality laughed nervously as he talked about having a drink in a bar with a professional football player who suddenly, and without explanation, pulled a knife on him. People cite that type of behavior when they talk about someone in the grip of what is called "roid rage."

Whether this phenomenon even occurs has been a subject of disagreement for years. Some experts point out that an entire generation of athletes used steroids without noticeably coming to public attention as criminally minded sociopaths. Many contemporary users take bigger doses for longer periods of time and in combination with other drugs, however, which may be a recipe for disaster. For example, a 20-year-old weight lifter beat a fellow bodybuilder to death after the victim made a pass at him in public. In another instance, a female steroid user beat her boyfriend so badly that he required medical treatment. There are reports in the literature of at least four other bodybuilders who were charged with murder or attempted murder during a period when they were abusing steroids.

There have now been a number of court cases in which the defendant's steroid abuse appeared to be a factor in the commission of a felony. Attorneys sometimes jokingly refer to the "roid rage" defense as the dumbbell defense. Diminished behavior control due to alcohol abuse also has been used as a defense in criminal cases, and juries have not shown themselves to be especially sympathetic to individuals who put themselves at risk by drinking. That appears to be the pattern for steroid-related diminished control as well. Unlike alcohol-induced personality changes that occur at the time alcohol is consumed, however, steroid-related personality changes take place over a longer period of time and may not be recognized or appreciated by the user. If behavior becomes violent and is clinically uncontrollable, then the level of intent becomes a real legal issue.

Although the "steroids made me do it" legal defense has been raised, more research is needed before the idea that steroids cause violent behavior in and of themselves will be widely accepted. Some steroid users may already be at the far end of a personality spectrum. In Dr. Bahrke's words, "It is probably safe to assume that individuals willing to take anabolic-androgenic steroids and other drugs of questionable origin, content, and purity, which have serious legal implications as well as health effects, differ from the population on a wide variety of characteristics, including mental health."

Indeed, a 1990 study of mental status changes in 20 competitive and noncompetitive weight lifters who used steroids found that they had more personality disturbances overall compared with a control group of 20 weight lifters who did not use steroids and a sex- and age-matched control group from the local community. Both the user and non-user weight lifters exhibited more flamboyant features (histrionic, narcissistic, antisocial, and borderline traits) when contrasted with the community controls. What behavioral alterations could be ascribed to steroids is unclear.

At this point, there is too much anecdotal evidence of uncontrollable aggression to discount entirely and too little research data to support a claim that steroid use will invariably cause uncontrolled aggression and hostility. Enough former steroid users are now serving prison time for offenses that featured out-of-control behavior that we should be concerned about the possibility of a connection, however.

COMMENTS BY DR. Y

In addition to helping to maintain order and protect the public safety, a country's laws serve as a moral compass. Legalizing steroids or any other illicit drug would send a terrible message to our citizens, especially to young people. However, a country that relies solely on laws to maintain order is in trouble. A society rises or falls with the values of its people. No amount of laws will maintain order in a society devoid of a strong ethical core.

Likewise in sport, rules define the game. But if the participants are devoid of a sense of fair play and sportsmanship, no set of rules can guarantee a clean contest. If a football coach teaches his offensive lineman to hold defensive players in a manner that the officials won't see, is he really a credible voice against steroid use in sport? Perhaps it's only cheating if you get caught. If sport is a microcosm of our society, isn't steroid use simply another example of societal decay?

My coauthor has strong feelings about this issue. Here is what she says: However imperfect our present systems might be, it would be a terrible mistake to consider legalizing performance-enhancing drugs. One need look no further than bodybuilding to see how widespread drug use has created a grotesque "ideal" image, acute serious medical crises, and even death, as the use of diuretics has. We cannot depend on athletes making judicious use of steroids during their athletic careers.

From the earliest times, the pattern has always been one of excess. Alcohol regulation does not entirely prevent alcohol abuse by youngsters but it serves as a check that is in the best interests of society.

CHAPTER 8

TREATMENT PROGRAMS

What happens when it's time to stop taking steroids? This matter is of great interest and concern because it now appears that some individuals may not be able to quit taking steroids without help. Almost all of the first wave of steroid users were athletes who took steroids to enhance their athletic performance. They took lower doses and fewer cycles of drugs than many of today's users and usually report that they simply stopped when their athletic careers were over.

For many current users, their body image is tied to their use of steroids. An athlete who uses steroids is already in good physical shape with musculature developed by hard work. Someone who has tried to take a shortcut by using steroids to develop a muscular and lean body may find a significant portion of the gains are lost when he discontinues steroids and their effects wear off. In some cases, this result provides a stimulus to keep using steroids.

The addictive potential of anabolic steroids has been a subject of discussion among experts for years. Some believe that what users are addicted to is the change in physical appearance or the enhancement of athletic performance. A few experts have theorized that steroids can be physically addictive and that they may cause physical withdrawal symptoms when a user discontinues taking them. While this academic debate goes on, some steroid users are simply struggling to stop.

Here are the words of one bodybuilder who got caught in an unending cycle of drug taking:

> When faced with the syringe, even my own worst fears didn't matter; I couldn't stop. Seventeen-inch arms were not enough, I wanted 20. And when I got to 20, I was sure that I'd want 22. My retreat to the weight room was a retreat into the simple world of numbers. Numerical gradations were the only thing left in my life that made sense. Twenty was better than 17 but worse than 22. Bench pressing 315 was better than bench pressing 275, but worse than 365. I was reduced to a world where such thinking ruled, and it was only by embracing it that I could sleep at night.

Such a powerful compulsion very likely requires professional help to get the person's life back on track.

Within the past several years, a consensus seems to have emerged that although anabolic steroids are not addictive in the same sense that cocaine or heroin is addictive, they are often abused substances, and some users do have trouble stopping. "What usually is meant in speaking of abuse is that some people use steroids in ways that the majority of people disapprove of," according to Kirk Brower, MD, a University of Michigan psychiatrist who has treated steroid users who were unable to stop on their own. He notes that in either the social or ethical sense, there is certainly reason to disapprove of using steroids for nonmedical uses, particularly the enhancement of sports performance. Nor, obviously, could society condone using powerful hormones with known negative health effects merely to improve physical appearance.

A major problem for steroid treatment at present and for the immediate future is a lack of funding. The money to study whether steroids have an addictive potential and to set up treatment programs simply is not there. With the cycle of recreational drug use moving into a new high point, most institutions and mental health professionals will be working with users of drugs that have high addictive potential, such as heroin, cocaine, crack, and amphetamines.

DEPENDENCE

In classic drug addiction, changes within the brain and body cause a craving for the abused drug, and physical withdrawal symptoms occur when use is discontinued. For instance, cocaine produces dependence through a mechanism called "primary reinforcement." Taking the drug stimulates the parts of the brain that are involved with reward, and a user feels pleasure or euphoria.

Although steroids don't appear to produce that type of immediate high, many users do say they feel pleasure from using the drugs over a period of time. The "high" they feel just occurs over a longer period of time. The knotty question then is whether they feel the high because the brain was stimulated or because they get a lot of pleasure from being stronger, having a big muscular body, or experiencing success in athletics. Some researchers have reported mood elevation in patients who were taking steroids for medical reasons, but it is still unclear whether steroids can cause the type of physical and/or psychological dependence that occurs with cocaine use.

We do know that anabolic steroids enter the brain and become attached to certain receptor sites. One study demonstrated that steroids can affect the same neurotransmitters that are involved in the action of cocaine and other stimulants on the brain. If steroids do have the potential to cause physical dependence, educational programs or penalties alone would not be enough to turn an addicted user away from the drugs.

Even though steroids have been in use for more than 50 years, scientists have focused most of their efforts in documenting their physical effects. Only within the last decade has concern grown that steroids may have a profound effect on mood and behavior in addition to their negative effects on physical health. The area of mood and behavior has the most potential for drug dependence. Most investigators now agree that steroids, especially at high doses, apparently can increase aggressiveness, but the studies in the medical literature are not uniform in this conclusion. Because most steroid users begin taking steroids for their effects on the body, they may not be fully aware of the possible mood-altering properties as well.

One particular matter of ongoing debate is the existence of what is popularly called "roid rage." This colorful term refers to spontaneous, highly aggressive, out-of-control violent behavior of a magnitude that the police are or should be involved. Although several scientists and many users claim to have observed steroid-induced episodes of uncontrolled violent behavior, others have questioned whether these episodes occurred and whether steroids were the cause.

One factor that may bear on roid rage and perhaps even addiction is that current users often take high doses and use different combinations of drugs together. Dosing schemes may have some effect on mood and behavior. Steroid users are also more likely to use other behavior-affecting drugs such as alcohol, cocaine, and amphetamines.

Certain characteristics distinguish heavy users who are at greatest risk for steroid dependence. They are more likely to have begun using steroids before age 16, to have completed more and longer drug cycles, to have combined multiple steroids simultaneously, and to have used injectable drugs. They are also more likely to perceive their peers as steroid users.

Criteria for Drug Dependency

The experts say that there is some evidence that steroids can lead to dependence. The next step then is to examine that evidence and define *dependence*. Psychiatrists are very specific in their definitions of "psychoactive substance dependence" caused by using drugs that alter mood, thinking, or behavior. To meet the psychiatric criteria for drug dependency, a user must have at least three of the following symptoms for at least one month before a diagnosis of substance-dependency is made:

- Takes more of the substance than intended
- Wants to stop or cut down use but is unable to do so
- Spends a lot of time on substance-related activity
- Is frequently intoxicated or suffering from withdrawal symptoms when expected to function or when physically hazardous
- Replaces social, work, or leisure activities with drug use
- Continues drug use despite problems caused or worsened by use
- Exhibits tolerance
- Has withdrawal symptoms

■ Uses the substance to relieve or avoid withdrawal symptoms

A number of studies of bodybuilders who use steroids have shown that 25 percent to more than 50 percent exhibit attitudes and behaviors that meet these criteria and are indicative of dependence on these drugs. There have been reports that for many in bodybuilding, where physical development is the purpose of the activity, taking steroids is an integral part of the lifestyle and subculture.

Whatever views anyone may hold regarding the potential for steroid addiction, scientific discussion of the subject has no meaning to an individual user who finds himself unable to stop behavior that he knows is clearly causing harm. The question then becomes one of offering help appropriately. If we believe that steroids produce dependence, we need to understand the mechanism of how this dependence happens in order to prevent and treat it.

Dr. Brower says it is possible that there is a primary reinforcement mechanism, as there is with drugs such as cocaine, but that hypothesis is far from being confirmed. For one reason, if there were a primary reinforcement mechanism, surely it would be harder for elite athletes who use steroids for an edge at the top level of competition to stop using them quite as easily as the large majority appear to do.

Adding another facet to this already complex subject, it now appears that there may be at least two distinct groups of steroid users and that dependence issues may be different between the groups. The first group includes those who take steroids to achieve their competitive goals, much the same way they use strength training and conditioning, sport psychology, or, for that matter, protective equipment. When their competitive years end, so does the need for steroids and other "tools of the trade." This user group may also use recreational drugs both during and after competitive athletics.

The second group of steroid users includes individuals who are not driven by athletic competition but by an image of self that is inexorably tied to their physical capacities (bench press or squat, and so on) or their appearance (size of arms, chest, legs, or percent body fat). Because steroids can significantly improve both physical capacities and appearance, and because discontinuation of steroids results in a significant loss of these gains, there is an incentive for prolonged use (dependence). This second group of users, which includes many bodybuilders, is driven by appearance concerns and, as a consequence, tends to use steroids over a long period of time. Chronic steroid use has been observed even among bodybuilders in their 40s, 50s, and 60s.

More research is needed to examine the question of physical and/or psychological drug dependence, whether there is a primary reinforcement mechanism, and whether other drug use potentiates psychological problems in steroid users. A 1989 review of the hypothesis of anabolic steroid addiction concluded that some abusers may develop a previously unrecognized steroid hormone-dependent disorder. Further research is needed to confirm this hypothesis and others about steroid addiction. Again, a general lack of funding for steroid research has hampered scientific inquiry into dependence and treatment issues.

AN APPROACH TO TREATMENT

However steroid use begins, the fact is that very few steroid users seek formal medical treatment unless they are having significant physical or psychological problems. Rather than seeking professional care, many users quit taking drugs when they do experience unacceptable physical problems, mood changes, or inappropriate aggressiveness. Because of the fact that steroids are controlled drugs and most heavy users get them from nonmedical sources, individuals may fear the consequences if they seek professional help. Dr. Brower said that a user may not immediately reveal the extent of his use even when he does come in for treatment. There have been reports of psychosis, mania, panic attacks, and violent or aggressive behavior associated with steroid use. If a user has committed a crime during a period of uncontrolled behavior, he or she may have the added complication of legal problems. For all these reasons, most of those who are seen for treatment of dependence represent the extreme.

Once the condition is known, the next step is to identify how the drugs affect the user's psychological state, behavior, or mood. According to Dr. Brower, the known symptoms that can occur when steroids are discontinued could be considered part of a withdrawal syndrome. In addition to craving steroids, users say they experience fatigue, a decrease in sexual interest, depression, muscular pains, and headache.

Depression is the symptom that causes the most concern among professionals because thoughts of suicide or suicide attempts have been observed in steroid users. The majority of withdrawal symptoms are depressive in nature, in fact. In one of the first studies of the psychiatric effects of steroids, researchers found that 12 percent of steroid users suffered from clinical depression during the first three months after discontinuing use. The time between onset of depression and presentation for treatment was between 1 and 14 months. The appearance of symptoms varies from person to person, however. The depression that occurs with discontinuation of steroid use is not necessarily limited to the period right after the user stops taking them. Moreover, a depressed mood may be caused by many factors, not just withdrawal.

Dr. Brower says that the following signs are signals that help is needed.

- Agitated or retarded behavior that is consistent with manic or depressive disorders
- Moods such as euphoria, irritability, depression, or anxiety
- Fast changes in affect or a sudden shift in moods
- A slower thought process as a result of depression or rapid and disorganized thought processes as part of a manic state
- Suicidal or homicidal thoughts or grandiose thoughts that may progress to delusions
- Hallucinations

A person who is severely dependent probably would demonstrate many of these signs and also have marked social dysfunction. Dr. Brower had one patient who exhibited six of the nine dependency symptoms. This man, whose wife left him because of his steroid-associated temper outbursts, experienced suicidal thoughts during withdrawal from the drugs.

Medication and Hospitalization

Patients who experience uncontrolled aggressiveness may need to be treated with antipsychotic medications, at least initially. Hospitalization is an option, depending on the degree of the violent or aggressive behavior and whether the patient must be sedated or restrained in some way. Other strong indications for hospitalization are if the individual is suicidal or if he has been unable to stop using steroids during outpatient treatment.

Steroid users who are trying to stop but don't require hospitalization may still need drug treatment to handle withdrawal symptoms and to help them abstain from using steroids while supportive therapy is being given. The drugs that may be given to relieve symptoms or treat other disorders that are present along with the steroid abuse include antidepressants, nonsteroidal anti-inflammatory drugs (NSAIDs), or tranquilizers.

Antidepressants may be useful for treating symptoms such as depressed mood and nervousness. The therapeutic action of antidepressants is usually attributed to the way they affect transmitters in the brain. These are the same transmitters that are affected by steroids; although the exact mechanism of action is not known, the stimulation of receptors may help the user's mood while the body's hormonal levels adjust. Care must be taken to prescribe the right amount of antidepressants, however. Not only is there considerable overdose potential with some antidepressants, but the drugs also can have a negative influence on the heart symptoms some users experience. Dr. Brower believes that a patient should have measurements of cardiac function before taking antidepressants.

NSAIDs such as ibuprofen or naproxen are often used to make the patient more comfortable during the withdrawal period. Musculoskeletal pain is a common complaint of users, particularly in those who attempt to lift the same amount of weight off steroids as they did while taking the drugs. NSAIDs relieve pain but do not have much potential for abuse. In addition to the musculoskeletal pain, longer periods of recovery between physical workouts, a feeling of getting smaller, and a feeling of regression in athletic performance or appearance can leave a former user vulnerable to a depressed mood state. If discontinuation causes diminished strength and longer recovery time after exercise, former users should be encouraged to reassess the frequency, duration, and intensity of their physical workouts so as to avoid dangerous stress to muscle, tendons, and ligaments.

Patients who cannot make a commitment to be abstinent should not be given other drugs, including opiates, tranquilizers, or even NSAIDs because of the danger of drug interactions and also because adding other drugs can only continue an individual's problem with drug-taking behavior. There can be a risk in giving drugs to help with withdrawal symptoms in some patients because the prescribed drugs also may have potential for abuse or because the prescribed drug could have a secondary black market value. It is very important for the physician to be certain that the user is not also abusing other illicit substances because of the dangers of drug interactions that could cause further damage or even death. For these reasons, drug treatment of steroid withdrawal requires a great deal of caution and professional attention.

Dr. Brower noted that in treating other drug-related dependencies, a physician may sometimes withdraw the patient from the drug gradually over time. This technique is almost impossible to do with steroids, however. Because many users take much higher doses than could ever prescribed in a clinical practice, a doctor could not ethically justify giving a patient reduced but still excessively high doses of steroids.

Some rationale exists for giving steroid preparations during the period of readjustment. During withdrawal, steroid abusers have abnormally low serum testosterone because taking the hormone from an outside source causes the body to decrease its own natural production. If a substitution program appears feasible, Dr. Brower said the physician probably would want to choose a relatively short-acting steroid ester of testosterone. Some patients also respond to human chorionic gonadotropin, which is a substance that stimulates the body to produce its own hormones.

Again, he cautions that writing a prescription for an abused substance to a substance abuser is not a good idea. Therefore, when a physician decides to substitute an ester of testosterone during the withdrawal period, he should administer the medication in his office or at a clinic. Take-home prescriptions should be avoided.

Dr. Brower notes that there haven't been studies to demonstrate that giving other drugs is helpful when a patient is discontinuing steroids, and he prefers a treatment plan of rapid discontinuation of the drugs, supportive therapy, and watchful waiting. He reserves other drug therapy and hospitalization for those whose symptoms are prolonged and severe or who may be suicidal or violent. There is a lack of clinical trials to help determine appropriate combinations of treatment for steroid dependence and withdrawal, and there also is a lack of physicians with experience in treating this type of drug abuse.

Importance of Supportive Therapy

Other supportive therapy may be needed to help a person discontinue use. Reassurance, education, and counseling are part of this therapy and should always be a part of the withdrawal process because of the risk of suicidal depression and relapse. Dr. Brower says a key to successful treatment is to establish a bond with the patient, and that bonding is most likely to occur when the patient views his doctor as nonjudgmental, knowledgeable about steroids and withdrawal, and understanding.

In Dr. Brower's view, the doctor should make it clear to the user that the decision to discontinue steroids is based on health concerns. Moral reasons are unlikely to have any impact on a steroid user's thinking at that point. Likewise, if the physician denies the benefits of steroids, the patient will see him as uninformed or disingenuous, and the physician will lose credibility, at the very least.

The physician or other health professional treating a steroid user must be able to see the situation through the eyes of the user, Dr. Brower believes. A doctor cannot be an effective therapist if he does not understand that the individual he is treating for steroid withdrawal perceives his reasons for taking steroids as rational. For instance, physical attributes and body image are a major source of concern to a bodybuilder; therefore, a psychotherapist who understands this point of view is more likely to help his patient find an acceptable alternative to steroids to maintain his body image.

Other potentially acceptable alternatives might include working with a nutritionist or exercise physiologist to achieve some of the goals that were first attained through drug use. The patient must be told that, if he continues with an exercise regimen, a significant amount of steroid-induced gains will be retained without the drugs. In addition, the patient must be encouraged to adopt more realistic goals related to strength and appearance. Ignoring the patient's unrealistic strength and appearance goals could condemn the treatment process to failure.

Dr. Brower advises being frank with patients about which withdrawal symptoms they are likely to experience, such as depression, so that if a symptom occurs, it isn't as frightening as it would be if it were unexpected. When patients anticipate symptoms and recognize them as part of the withdrawal from drugs, and not something wrong with themselves, they are better able to handle the frustrations and depressive moods that frequently occur during withdrawal.

The doctor should continue a process of education about steroids during therapy. The simple step of going over the abnormal physical state or laboratory tests with the patient reinforces the notion that discontinuation is part of a process of regaining good health. Some patients may want to keep track as some of the reversible abnormalities like testicular shrinkage or cholesterol levels become more nearly normal. Monitoring liver function during withdrawal is important, both as a measure of regaining health and because the state of the liver may have an impact on which drugs can be prescribed for muscle aches and pains.

Supportive therapy may be just a first step in learning to live without steroids. Some patients may need help to rebuild their lives after steroids. This process probably will include changing parts of their lives that were associated with their drug use—perhaps they need to change not only where they exercise, but also change their circle of friends and reassess certain life goals and expectations. Because steroid use can be so intricately woven into a user's lifestyle, psychological counseling may be an important step in discontinuing use.

COMMENTS BY DR. Y

Assessing the behavioral effects of anabolic steroids has been mired in controversy, in part due to the sensationalistic way the news media has handled this topic. For example, several years ago, a popular magazine interviewed me about a young man whose life was in great turmoil because of his steroid use. This young man acknowledged that before he ever took his first steroid, he did not "fit in" at school, he abused alcohol, and he was physically abusive of his mother. During his period of steroid use, he also used IV amphetamines and was admitted to a hospital because of a Valium overdose. Therefore, imagine my surprise when the author of the article concluded that all of his problems stemmed from his steroid abuse. While the premise is silly, it is an example of the fact that steroid items in the popular media can be long on sensationalism and short on scientific fact.

What is the bottom line on steroids and behavior? I believe that steroids do indeed make you more aggressive. Although most users will be able to control these increased aggressive urges and not get in serious trouble with the law, a few will not. The real bad news is that the prospective user can't look in the mirror and tell whether he or she will be one of those that could go over the edge and land in serious trouble. Still more to the point, even if a teenager is not in that group, does he or she need to take hormones that can adversely change mood and behavior during a time in their life when their natural hormone levels are already presenting them with enough challenges?

People often ask me: can you get hooked on steroids? I think so, especially if the primary motivation for use is to become more muscular, and how you look and how much weight you can lift are very important to you. I have seen too many cases where a young man says he is only going to use steroids for one cycle to gain 15 pounds. He does that and finds it wasn't that difficult, so he decides to go for another 15 pounds, reasoning: "Maybe I'll take just one more cycle." And it goes on and on. When he finally stops using steroids, some, but not all, of the muscle and strength gains are lost. His chest, arms, and legs are not quite as big or defined, and his bench press and squat weights have dropped. He notices, and some of his friends notice too. Well, just one more cycle won't hurt—will it? That way lies addiction.

ALTERNATIVES, PROBLEMS, AND IDEAS

The problems that steroids cause, both to the individual and to sports and society, have now been stated. The strategies being used to combat steroid use have been explained. It is obvious that there is work to be done. There are several reasons why only varying degrees of success have been achieved over the years. Perhaps first and foremost is the fact that a large segment of society looks to drugs to supply what they need. Second is the fact that many people simply do not see a connection between taking drugs and cheating.

For instance, a young mother was overheard at a swim meet confiding to a friend her happiness that the pediatrician had put her daughter on steroids because it would improve her swim times. She was, of course, confused; it was an asthma medication, a corticosteroid, that had been supplied and not anabolic steroids. But her daughter was under the age of 10, and already the idea of taking drugs to enhance performance was present.

The good news is that there are ways to maximize performance that are ethical, legal, and good for you in that they have lasting health benefits. Conversation with Olympians at the 1996 Games in Atlanta convinces both of us that athletes prefer clean contests. Having spent years developing a skill to the very highest peak, they are looking to test themselves against the world's best athletes, not the world's best chemists. A majority of Olympic athletes appear to be strong proponents of drug testing because of their desire to maintain sports as a manifestation of human excellence.

Offering sound alternatives to drug use from the outset is important. Proper strength training and good nutrition can help athletes improve performance immensely, but most people don't know how to get started or how to judge either a conditioning program or a sports-specific diet. The ATLAS program has shown the way, providing sound grounding in weight training and nutrition in combination with a steroid education program. It has demonstrated that young athletes who are soundly grounded in ways to maximize their physical potential will not feel as much need to look to pills and potions. Because the topics of nutrition and strength training are so important, we are including chapters by two experts in these fields in this section of the book.

In order to improve our current lines of defense, we must scrutinize them carefully for weaknesses so that they can be strengthened and revised, if necessary. Drug testing is our main line of defense at the elite level and likely to remain so, even if it is not the complete answer. We know, for instance, that there is no test as yet for two effective substances that are popular with athletes, erythropoietin and human growth hormone. Erythropoietin (EPO) was developed to stimulate the body to produce more red blood cells and is a legitimate medical treatment for anemia. However, having more red blood cells in the body means more oxygen is transported to working muscles and aerobic capacity improves. EPO has largely replaced blood doping, a complicated procedure that involves blood transfusions and that can increase the risk of disease transmission.

Human growth hormone (hGH) regulates a number of processes in the human body, and a synthetic hGH has been on the market since the mid 1980s. It, too, has legitimate medical uses; a deficiency or absence of this vital hormone results in dwarfism. However, hGH quickly found a black market use among athletes who like it because it helps build muscle and shed fat. Neither EPO or hGH has quite the same type of adverse health effects as anabolic steroids, although both can be dangerous in excess.

There are a number of serious problems with the process of drug testing despite the fine work done in the IOC-approved drug testing laboratories. Although athletes who are caught cheating often protest that a mistake was made in the laboratory, in actual fact, the United States IOC-approved drug testing laboratories are without peer. The samples are carefully analyzed, and if there is a positive test, a second sample is analyzed. But drug testing has a political as well as a technical component, and the political element needs significant refinement and improvement.

Of course, not all steroid use occurs among athletes. No significant progress has been made toward reducing the number of users in the general population who often have nothing to do with organized sports. Elite military units, firefighters, and police, any occupation that requires strength and power or that is physically depleting, often include individuals who take anabolic steroids. What harm this use may be doing, we don't know.

If testosterone becomes more accepted as an antidote for aging, a male contraceptive, or hormone replacement therapy, the distinction between legitimate and unethical use of hormones is likely to become difficult to make. Just as many postmenopausal women take estrogen replacement therapy, with the short-term evidence showing that there are protective effects, it may be that testosterone will be increasingly used to treat a variety of legitimate male health needs.

This use does not mean that it would be OK to use them in healthy youngsters to help them win at games. It may be that sports contests have become more important as the physical challenges that once were once part of everyday life in a less technologically developed era decreased. Whatever the cause, the effect has been developmentally unhealthy. Most experts would like to see an agreement reached about what is right and wrong behavior on the part of athletes and sports federations alike.

Part III is intended to give you information that can be used as a starting point to identify healthy ways of looking at sports performance in general and at the negative role drugs now play. Physical excellence would not continue to fascinate us if it did not meet some deeper human need. Therefore, protecting the physical expression of that excellence is a prudent investment in our future.

CHAPTER 9

STRENGTH TRAINING

William J. Kraemer, PhD
Center for Sports Medicine/Department of Kinesiology
The Pennsylvania State University

Some athletes are tempted to take anabolic drugs for better, faster results. They become frustrated when their strength training program doesn't quickly produce the enhanced fitness and appearance, the "buffed" look, of a trained body. Instead of trying to find a better training program, they opt for trying to achieve the desired results through the use of anabolic drugs.

A key part of prevention efforts is to help athletes understand that steroid-produced gains are not physiologically sound. The artificial drug approach relies on chemical manipulation instead of on maximizing the body's own natural anabolic output from the hormonal system. Gains in physical size and strength that are produced by steroids are "real," but some of the gains are lost after the drug is discontinued.

Conversely, an athlete who is patient, works hard, and understands basic training principles can make real, long-lasting improvements in appearance that will have positive physical and psychological effects for a lifetime. Strength training truly should be a lifetime pursuit, as it is strongly associated with health and fitness. Although the ability of athletes to adapt physiologically changes over the years from childhood to adulthood, the importance of strength training has been demonstrated in all age groups, from youth well into old age.

The keys to success with strength training are proper program design, progression, and supervision. The benefits of a sound, properly supervised training program include the following:

- Increased general muscular strength and local muscular endurance (for example, the ability of muscles to perform multiple repetitions against a given resistance)

- Prevention of injuries caused by the stress of participation in sports and recreational activities

- Improved performance capacity in sports and recreational activities

- Gains in muscle size (after adolescence and more pronounced in males) or gains in the quality muscle protein (all ages)

STRENGTH TRAINING TERMS

Here is a listing of basic terms and key concepts in strength training that you should know.

Term	Definition
barbell	A weight normally lifted with both arms
concentric	Shortening of a muscle during an exercise movement, typically when the resistance is being lifted
dumbbell	A weight normally lifted with only one arm
eccentric	Lengthening of a muscle during an exercise movement, typically when the resistance is being lowered
equipment fit	How the individual body (limb lengths, height) fits the resistance training apparatus
free weights	Barbells and dumbbells

frequency	Number of times per week one resistance exercise is performed
intensity	The resistance or weight used in an exercise
machines	Resistance training equipment where the equipment dictates the direction of the movement and position
progressive overload	Gradual increase in exercise stress (for example, increasing intensity)
proper breathing	Breathing out on the lifting movement and breathing in on the lowering part of the exercise
range of motion	Degree of movement permitted by joints and body position in a given exercise
repetition (rep)	Performance of one resistance exercise movement (for example, performing one arm curl)
repetition maximum (RM)	The maximum number of repetitions possible with a given intensity (for example, 1 RM, 5 RM, 10 RM)
set	A group of repetitions (for example, 3 sets of 10 repetitions)
specificity	Adaptations that occur in the muscle(s) used in response to a particular exercise
spotter	The individual responsible for the safety of the athlete performing a lift
variation	Changing intensity and volume (or other exercise variables such as rest periods) to provide a different stimulus
volume	Sets multiplied by repetitions multiplied by resistance equals volume

Parents, teachers, and coaches can play a major role in health and fitness by working together to see that programs are properly designed, correctly taught, and properly supervised.

ESTABLISHING PROPER TRAINING GOALS

The two major reasons why athletes may not achieve success with their strength training are lack of knowledge of how to design a strength training program and improper expectations. Both of these factors explain why some athletes fail to give natural resistance training methods enough time to work. It takes from six months to a year to get really visible results. Anyone who starts resistance training should be prepared to stick with the program for at least that length of time before deciding whether it is worthwhile.

Inappropriate training goals and objectives also lead to problems and failure. Unfortunately, the exaggerated body images popularized in the news, entertainment, and sports media often promote false assumptions about strength training. The positive benefits of a strength training program can get lost in the chase for the extreme in physical development. That image may bear little resemblance to the real benefits that can be obtained through a consistent and well-developed strength training program. The true goals of strength training are improved strength and power, improved muscular endurance, and improved quality and quantity of muscle (depending upon age). Remember and reinforce these goals so that the athlete's main emphasis is not on physical appearance.

TAILORING THE TRAINING PROGRAM

Successful progressive resistance programs are custom-made to the specific needs of the athlete. Even then, the program must be adjusted during the training period. Strength training is not a "one size fits all" activity. It is unrealistic to expect every individual doing strength training to proceed at the same pace. Sample programs can be used as a starting point, but specifics of any program and the rate of progression must be fitted to the individual response to training.

AGE-APPROPRIATE STRENGTH TRAINING

Parents and coaches are often unsure about young athletes' physical readiness for strength training. They may believe that it should be delayed until after puberty. The truth is that when children are physically capable of participating in a competitive sport, they are also capable of participating in a properly designed and supervised resistance training program. All of the major medical and scientific associations agree that resistance training can be very beneficial to children. Sports medicine and strength and conditioning professionals support resistance exercise programs for children so long as the program is properly designed, correctly taught, and adequately supervised.

Age	Recommended exercise
8 to 10	Start with little or no weight, gradually increase the number of exercises, and practice exercise technique in all lifts. Start gradual progressive loading of exercises, keep exercises simple, progress from low volume and carefully monitor toleration to the exercise stress.
11 to 13	Perform all basic exercise techniques, continue progressive loading of each exercise, and again emphasize exercise techniques. Introduce more advanced exercises with little or no resistance.
14 to 15	Progress to more advanced youth programs in resistance exercise, add sport-specific components, emphasize exercise techniques, and increase volume.
16 and older	Proceed to the entry level of adult programs after gaining the necessary background experience.

Note: When a child enters an age level with no previous experience in resistance training, progression must start at previous levels and move to more advanced levels as exercise toleration, skill, and understanding permits.

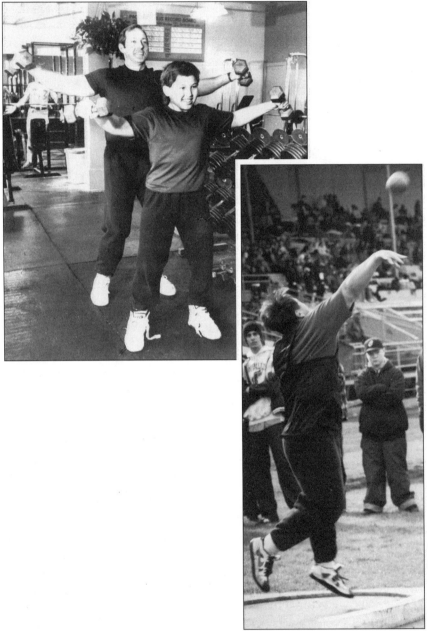

By age 10, Chris Sprague was lifting weights regularly with the careful supervision of his father, Ken and at age 16, Chris set a national record in the shot put with the effort shown here. Properly planned and executed training programs and coaching can help athletes achieve great feats.

Just as uniforms and athletic shoes must be fitted, so must an exercise program.

For example, consider the 300-pound bench press. Many freshmen football players believe this feat is a measure of real strength. Nothing is inherently wrong with that goal, but all 15-year-old football players cannot achieve it. Even more important is the fact that the bench press is not correlated with football success. The ability to bench press favors individuals with short arms and big chests, and these characteristics are genetically determined. Pressing this much weight at the age of 15 is almost impossible for a tall athlete with long arms and a shallow chest. Even an athlete with the right size dimensions might not have the necessary number of muscle fibers to attain that level of strength at age 15.

Still, many adolescent football players are confronted by a coach who barks, "If you want to make the team, you better get that bench press up there." This signal is wrong. Too much emphasis is put on one specific lift, the bench press. Moreover, the hidden message is that physical strength equates with football success (forgetting technique and understanding of strategy).

It is painfully obvious to most 15 year olds that a 300-pound bench press is not a realistic goal. A better goal is improvement in chest strength, without using arbitrary numbers. More important is adherence to training and development of the joy that comes with the challenge of physical activity.

DEVELOPING STRENGTH PROGRAMS AND WORKOUTS

Strength training programs must change as an individual matures and/or becomes more fit. Moreover, goals may change because of the demands of a particular phase of life. This systematic process of varying a strength training program has been called *periodization* of training. The purpose is to avoid overtraining, provide time for physical and mental recovery, and allow the athlete to make continued gains with a training program. Many systems of program periodization have been developed over the past 10 years, and it appears that the key to the general concept is based in the need for variation of the workout stimulus.

The challenge to any long-term training program is adherence to

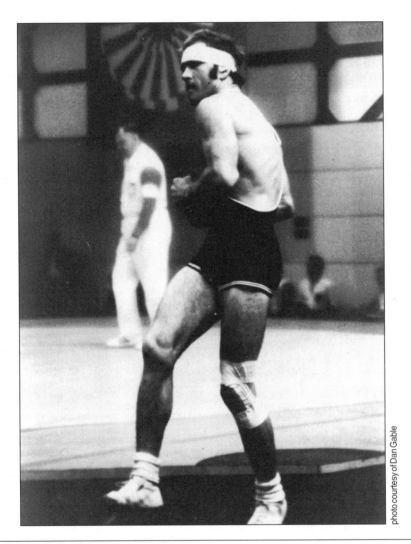

photo courtesy of Dan Gable

One of the greatest competitors in the history of sports, Dan Gable's mental toughness and focus enabled him to use his superior conditioning and technical skills to dominate the 1972 Olympics without allowing an opponent a single point.

the program and keeping it effective. When a training program never changes, a program becomes boring, and the individual ceases to look forward to a workout. One solution to this problem that might encourage long-term adherence to a program in children is to use periodized strength training.

You can achieve periodized training in several ways by altering workout variables such as the choice of exercise, order of exercise, or amount of rest between sets and exercises. This section focuses on how you might alter the intensity and volume (sets multiplied by repetitions multiplied by resistance) of a core group of large muscle group exercises, such as the squat/leg press, bench press, seated rows, military press, and lat pulldown.

Typically, the larger muscle group exercises are periodized, but all exercises can be varied for intensity. One method is to vary intensity over the week, for example, Monday (light), Wednesday (heavy), and Friday (moderate), for a given training period (usually 8 to 12 weeks) before competition is started or an active rest (activity but not lifting) is allowed. Then the training program goes into a new 8 to 12 week cycle. Another method of periodization of training varies the intensity over several weeks (or cycles) of training, for example, Weeks 1 to 4 (light), Weeks 5 to 8 (moderate), and Weeks 9 to 12 (heavy). Usually the number of weeks used is called a *microcycle* and ranges from 2 to 4 weeks.

After the last cycle or at the end of a training period, competitions are usually scheduled because the athlete is at his or her peak for that period of training. Or the athlete can enter into an in-season program where he or she lifts once or twice a week to maintain gains. The first method of variation is usually preferred so that training can continue through the season. This continued training is especially important for sports with long seasons (such as tennis, wrestling, basketball, and hockey).

The key element of this type of training is the variation and ability to allow rest after a training or competition period. Strength can be maintained easier than it can be gained, so periods of active rest allow the athlete to stay active but not necessarily lift weights. The length of active rest is related to the amount of training the athlete has had and where the rest is taken in the yearly cycle. Usually active rest ranges from one to four weeks in adults, with the less-experienced athletes taking the shorter one to two week breaks before a new cycle of training begins.

Evidence suggests that variation in exercises for the same muscle group causes greater increases in strength and power than no variation in exercises. This evidence does not mean that the exercises performed must be changed every single training session or that all exercises must be changed when one change is made. You can make changes in exercises every two to three weeks or vary some exercises on an every other training session basis and perform two somewhat different training sessions alternately.

For example, the exercise included for the arms and shoulder might be the bench press, which is changed to the incline press or a bench press with dumbbells at two- to three-week intervals. You could make these same changes on alternate training sessions. For example, on Monday and Friday, you could do the bench press, and on Wednesday, you could do the incline press. You should maintain certain core exercises throughout the training program for optimum progress, however.

Phase-by-Phase Strength Program

■ **General pre-preparation phase.** This period of six to eight weeks is used for general strength conditioning to allow the athlete to tolerate the strength training program. Stress correct exercise technique with little or no resistance. Start out at a low intensity that permits at least 12 to 15 repetitions. Start with a low volume of exercise by using only one or two sets and a low number of exercises. Add exercises as the athlete learns how to properly perform the exercises. Large muscle group exercises are usually periodized, and small muscle group exercises (such as arm curls and leg curls) are performed with a moderate intensity (8 to 10 repetitions max, or RM). Nevertheless, you can periodize these exercises in a similar manner as the large muscle group exercises.

The number of times through the training cycle phases is determined by the amount of time before the season. Several cycles are probably better than one large one, and thus, the length of each phase has been reduced to as little as two-week cycles. Typically, a minimum of six weeks is allowed for the three cycle phases to be completed. Training is usually done three times a week.

■ **Preparation phase.** Choose a cycle length from two to four weeks that will be used for all of the following lift cycles. This phase formally starts a training cycle, and the number of exercises and initial toleration should be in place from the prior cycle. Perform two to three sets of each exercise at an intensity that allows between 12 and 15 repetitions. This level of intensity creates a high-volume, low-intensity stimulus. There is a one- to two-minute rest period between sets and exercises.

■ **Power phase.** Using the same length cycle of two to four weeks, the individual uses a resistance that allows only 8 to 10 repetitions and performs two to three sets of each exercise. Rest periods of one and a half to two minutes come between sets and exercises. Again, technique is stressed, along with progression in the resistance that can be used for the repetitions performed.

■ **Strength phase.** Using the same length cycle of two to four weeks, the resistance used now allows only 6 or 7 repetitions. The athlete does two or three sets of each exercise, with two to two and a half-minute rest periods between sets and exercises. Technique is stressed as well as progression in the resistance that can be used for the repetitions performed.

■ **Transition phase**. After the athlete moves into the competitive sport season, initiate an in-season program. The workout may vary among heavy, light, and moderate intensities, as used in the other method of periodized training mentioned later in the chapter. The key is to maintain strength and power but reduce the total amount of exercise.

Nonlinear Strength Program

Start with a general pre-preparation phase identical to the one described previously. This nonlinear method uses 8 to 12 week cycles of training where on different days the athlete uses a light (12 to 15 repetitions, 2 to 3 sets, 1 to 2 minutes of rest), heavy (6 to 7 RM, 2 to 3 sets, 2 to 3 minutes of rest), or a moderate (8 to 10 RM, 2 to 3 sets, 1.2 to 2 minutes of rest) program. The thought is that varying the workout within the week provides adequate recovery and variation. At the end of a training cycle, an athlete enters an in-season program using the same method of intensity variation but with a reduced number of exercises or sets to lower the volume of training.

Strength Training Workouts

A strength training program consists of well-planned individual and weekly workout regimens. Consider these variables when developing workouts:

■ **Choice of exercise.** Choose resistance exercises that work all of the major muscle groups in the body. Make sure you exercise each side of a joint (for example, the front [biceps] and back [triceps] of the arm) and perform both upper body (bench press) and lower body (squat) exercises. The equipment should fit your body dimensions;

some machines are made for the normative male. When in doubt, use free weights, which fit any body size.

■ **Order of exercises.** Typically an athlete performs large muscle group exercises or more complex exercises at the beginning of a workout. Move from arm to leg exercises if you're using a circuit program.

■ **Number of sets.** Begin with one set of each exercise; as adaptation occurs, progress to three sets of each exercise in a program.

■ **Intensity of exercise.** A maximum load (RM) of six repetitions is what is typically recommended for prepubescent children. As an athlete moves into adolescence (age 15 or 16) he or she can use heavier loads. Usually training zones are used as targets; for example, a target load of 6 to 8 repetitions or a load of 10 to 12 repetitions. You don't need to squeeze out the very last repetition just to make sure that the load has enough repetitions in the target range to achieve the expected adaptations. More strength will be gained with the use of a 6 to 8 RM than with a 12 RM. Thus loading intensity determines the strength gains made in young athletes.

■ **Rest between sets and exercises.** Rest periods should be 3 minutes or more when heavier resistances (1 to 6 RM) are used, 2 to 3 minutes with moderate (7 to 10 RM) resistances, and 1 to 2 minutes when lighter resistances (11 RM or greater) are used. Nevertheless, the rest period should last until the athlete feels ready to lift the weight safely. Short rest periods (less than 2 minutes) are more stressful and are indicated only if the athlete can tolerate the metabolic demands and has gradually progressed to the lower rest level over a training period.

After those five variables are addressed, the next issue is how to make progress over a period of time. Progress usually involves some type of periodization or program variation. A strength training program that never varies soon becomes boring and ineffective. Enthusiasm for training is likely to wane, and there may be a loss of physical benefits gained if training is stopped. A systematic variation of strength training program variables (such as intensity of the exercise) is extremely important.

Motivation and Program Philosophy

Every program, whether it is a home fitness program, school athletic program, private health club, or public recreation facility needs to make the environment conducive to training. This task requires developing and implementing a program philosophy with motivational considerations and realistic program expectations.

Providing the right motivation for athletes is a very individual phenomenon that should always be viewed from a trainee's perspective. The first step is getting the athletes genuinely interested in physical fitness. Don't use the exercise program as punishment for unwanted behaviors such as missing a catch or free throw. When used this way, exercise becomes a negative thing.

Another mistake happens when coaches or parents overshoot a youngster's physical capabilities and make the experience physically painful. One example is having the individual perform drills or exercise routines that are inappropriate from the standpoint of an exercise prescription. Performing too many sets during the first training sessions of a program also may result in severe muscle soreness and take away from the enjoyment of the physical activity. With proper progression, each athlete will be prepared physically and mentally for sports participation.

As anabolic steroids and other alternatives become even more widely available, promoting fitness activities in a positive way is even more important. Properly conducted resistance training can help prepare athletes for sports or help people enjoy better physical health. Strength training is a great activity, one of the primary interventions that can help the body develop naturally. When its basic principles are understood, they are likely to reduce or limit the temptation to use anabolic drugs for physical development.

STRENGTH TRAINING SAFELY

The potential for injury is one of the biggest concerns about strength training. In reality, the incidence of strength training injuries is very low and is far less than the ever-increasing frequency of sports-related injuries in athletes, some of which are caused by playing a sport while out of shape. The notion that athletes can "play themselves into shape" has been proven false many times, but still too many athletes start a sports season without proper conditioning. Injury is far less likely when strength training is used as a conditioning tool to enable athletes to handle the physical demands of sports.

Patience and knowledge are prerequisites for teaching or performing strength training exercise techniques. Lack of knowledge and improper lifting and spotting techniques are the primary causes of injury. Don't rush, and be sure to emphasize correct exercise techniques for a safe and effective program.

Proper Exercise Technique

The first step in being able to teach or perform resistance exercises is to know proper exercise techniques (see references at end of book for further reading). Regardless of the source of the information, the strength trainer should be sure he or she completely understands the technique of the exercise before attempting to teach it. This requirement is especially important for multijoint exercises, such as the squat. An effective teacher will take the time to study and practice the lifts.

When learning a new exercise, start with very light resistance. Critique the exercise technique or have an experienced individual do a critique. This critique will help you learn proper exercise technique as quickly as possible and is one reason for having a training partner. Correct exercise technique is mandatory for doing resistance exercises properly.

Proper technique means performing the exercise with the fullest possible range of movement dictated by the body position of the exercise and with only those muscles that are supposed to be involved. Full range of motion means lowering and lifting the resistance over the desired distance. In some exercises, for safety considerations, you can set the range of motion (for example, only half-squats, or 30-degree arc knee extensions, or benching to two inches above the chest). Improper exercise technique causes muscles

STRENGTH TRAINING CHECKLIST

To prevent injury while training, follow these guidelines:
- Use a properly designed and supervised program
- Know how to perform the exercise and use the equipment
- Have proper spotting during the exercise
- Do not hold your breath when performing an exercise
- Go through the full range of motion

that are not supposed to be trained by the exercise to be used. This improper technique compromises the training effect for those muscles that the exercise was supposed to train.

Poor exercise technique may also cause undue stress on a body part and result in injury. This possibility is especially prevalent in exercises involving the lower back, especially when there is heavy resistances, such as with squats or dead lifts. The lower back can also be injured during such exercises as arm curls and the shoulder press if a rocking motion of the back is used to initiate movement of the resistance.

Improper progression in resistance is another way that injury can occur. Often, this improper progression is because the increases in resistance are too great or occur too soon in the training program. Proper exercise programming and technique can prevent most resistance training injuries.

Proper Spotting Technique

Knowing how to properly spot the exercise is as important as knowing proper exercise technique, and it is vital to a safely conducted resistance training program. No one should lift alone at any time. Both the supervisor and all athletes should know correct exercise and spotting techniques for all exercises performed in the training program. Spotters can aid the injury prevention effort by correcting any errors in lifting technique. Also, spotters must be strong enough to aid the trainee if necessary. Spotters should know

SPOTTING CHECKLIST

A good spotter meets these criteria:

- Knows proper exercise technique
- Is strong enough to assist the lifter with the resistance being used if needed
- Knows how many repetitions the lifter intends to do
- Is attentive to the lifter at all times
- Corrects the lifter's technique when wrong
- Knows the plan of action if a serious injury occurs

how many repetitions are being attempted, and they must be attentive to the lifter at all times.

Number of Exercises

Attempting to learn too many exercises at once, especially multijoint exercises, is counterproductive. The number of exercises an individual can learn proper technique for at one time will vary. Start with seven or eight exercises, of which one to three may be multijoint exercises.

Proper Breathing Technique

Proper breathing for resistance training exercises means inhaling just before and during the lowering phase of the lift and exhaling during the lifting phase of the repetition. When isometric training is performed, it is important that the breath is not held during the muscular contraction. During the last repetition of a set or during heavy lifts (such as 1 to 6 RM), some breath holding will occur, but breath holding throughout a complete repetition should not be allowed.

Blood pressure rises dramatically with breath holding, called a Valsalva maneuver. This rise in blood pressure makes it very difficult for the heart to pump blood and reduces blood flow back to the heart from the rest of the body. Moreover, blood flow to the head and brain is reduced when the breath is released. This reduction can cause a light-headed feeling after completion of a set, even fainting. Should fainting occur, there could be a loss of control of the resistance, possibly leading to injury. Because maximal or near maximal resistances are not the object for a young trainee, excessive breath holding should not be allowed.

Slow Increase in Resistance

Increasing the resistance too quickly slows down the learning process for acquiring good technique and could result in injury. A good guideline to follow is that when an increase of resistance results in poor technique, the increase was too great at that point in the training program. This guideline is true for both beginning and experienced lifters.

During the initial three to four weeks of a resistance training program, large increases in the resistance that can be used are typical. Smaller increases in the resistances that can be used occur at the start of a training program if the individual has previously performed the exercise. These increases do not represent true increases in strength or power; instead, they demonstrate that the individual has learned to perform the exercise correctly.

These initial large increases in the resistance that can be lifted have several implications, however. First, testing to evaluate the present strength or power of an individual should not be done until the exercise can be properly performed. Second, the magnitude of the initial increases will be less with an individual who has previously resistance trained. This information is needed to set realistic goals for increases in strength due to the training program.

Symmetrical Muscular Development

Another important point to consider is the use of unilateral exercises (single arm or leg exercises versus two-arm or two-leg exercises). Examples of unilateral exercises are the lunge, which exercises one leg at a time; single-leg knee extensions and knee curls on a machine, which allows performance of the exercise using one leg at a time; and a one-arm shoulder press with dumbbells. Conversely, a leg press and bench press using both legs or both arms at the same time are examples of bilateral exercises.

Symmetrical development is dependent upon using single arm and leg exercises. When only double arm or leg (bilateral) exercises are used, the stronger limb can compensate for the weaker one. This situation is especially true on most resistance training machines. Although it is natural for one arm or leg to be stronger, proper exercise programming and use of unilateral exercises can reduce any drastic differences. Ideally, the difference in strength between limbs should be less than 10 percent. The similarity in strength between limbs helps promote good physical development and reduces the possibility of injury. Although bilateral exercises are important, the use or choice of appropriate unilateral exercises must be given consideration, especially in programs for the physical development of youngsters.

Muscle balance around a joint is also very important. Thus, if one does a quad exercise (front of upper leg) during a workout, then that

SAFETY FIRST

Of all the sport and recreational activities, strength training has one of the lowest incidences of injury. In general, it is a safe activity. The potential for injury is there, however, and the following are some possible causes of injury:

- Attempting to lift a resistance that is too heavy
- Improper lifting technique
- Improper placement of feet or hands on a resistance training machine so they slide off the pedals or handles of the machine
- Placing hands on the chain or pulley system of a resistance training machine
- Placing hands between the weight plates of a resistance training machine
- Dropping free weights or the weight stack of a resistance training machine after completion of a repetition
- Inattentive spotters
- Improper behavior in the facility
- A bench or piece of equipment sliding during the exercise
- Worn out equipment that breaks during lifting (for example, machine cables or pulleys)
- Collars not used on free weights
- Accidental dropping of free weight plates while loading or unloading a bar

person should also do a hamstring (back of upper leg) exercise. Promoting balance of the muscle around a joint may reduce the potential for injury.

Machines or Free Weights?

The controversy over whether resistance machines or free weights produce the greatest gains in strength and power probably started right after the first resistance machine was invented. Machines allow movement only in a predetermined plane and path of movement, so balancing the resistance in all directions is not necessary. The need to balance the resistance with free weights requires the use of muscles not involved in the movement as prime movers.

For instance, prime movers in the military press are the outside of the shoulder area (deltoid) and the back of the upper arm (triceps). The muscles of the upper and lower back, smaller muscles around the shoulder area, and even the abdominal muscles are involved in balancing the resistance, however. The involvement of these secondary or balancing muscles is greater with free weights than machines. Advocates of free weights claim the need to balance the resistance is more like what occurs in sports events or in daily life where balancing of any resistance moved is necessary.

Conversely, machine advocates claim that not having to balance a resistance is good because it allows greater isolation of the muscles involved in the exercise as prime movers. They also claim that teaching proper technique is easier because movement is allowed only in one plane and direction. Both sides in this controversy use the same facts but interpret them to be positive from their particular point of view. This controversy may be confusing for others and can lead to confusion when decisions about equipment are being made.

In reality, the strengths or weaknesses of machines or free weights can all be used to advantage in a resistance training program. Machines do allow movement in only one plane and direction, and the isolation of a muscle group is very useful when the goal of the program is to increase strength or power or the local muscular endurance of a specific muscle group. This feature makes them ideal for rehabilitation after an injury. Machines are also very good when the goal is to increase strength and power or local muscular endurance for a particular muscle group or joint that is prone to injury in a particular sport or in a muscle group that is the weak link in performance of a certain sporting activity. Free weight exercises, which require you to balance the resistance, are a good choice when the goal is to strengthen total body movements and provide coordination between various muscle groups. Thus, both machine (fixed form) and free weight (free form) exercises have a place in a well-designed resistance training program.

There are two other matters to be addressed regarding free weights and machine exercises. Although the research is not conclusive, adult free weight exercises such as squats, appear to provide greater increases in vertical jumping ability than performing machine leg press exercises. This difference may be because squats have a greater mechanical similarity to the jumping motion. Both squat and leg press type exercises can increase vertical jumping ability, however. The second matter concerns exercise technique. A greater amount of time needs to be planned to teach free weight exercises because of the need to balance the weight.

Despite the claims of equipment manufacturers, research has shown virtually all resistance training equipment gives essentially equal gains in strength and power and motor performance tests. (The 40-yard sprint and maximal vertical jump are common motor performance tests.) One interpretation is that gains in strength and power and motor performance are more dependent upon the design of the training program and upon the effort the individual puts into the program than upon the type of equipment.

When you must make decisions about purchasing or using various pieces of equipment, consider these factors:

- If the equipment does not fit the athlete, can it be safely altered to do so?
- If you are purchasing the equipment, what is its cost per exercise station?
- If purchasing the equipment, how much will it cost to purchase sufficient equipment to perform an exercise for all major muscle groups of the body?
- If you are purchasing the equipment, how long is its warranty?
- If you are purchasing the equipment, what does its warranty cover?
- Is the equipment made from heavy gauge steel?
- Is the equipment sturdily constructed (for example, are the welds solid)?
- How easy is it to adjust the resistance?
- Does the resistance increase in increments suitable for children?

FOR FURTHER READING ON THIS TOPIC

For more complete information on strength training, including program design principles, sport-specific programs, exercise spotting and lifting techniques, and safety tips, consult the books in the Suggested Readings on page 196 of this book.

CHAPTER 10

WHAT IS GOOD SPORTS NUTRITION?

Nancy Clark, MS, RD
SportsMedicine Brookline

A more healthful way to enhance sports performance and achieve some of the gains athletes look for when they take anabolic steroids is to practice good sports nutrition. Food is fuel. The right foods enhance performance; the wrong ones hurt performance. Most elite athletes learn to manage their food intake as a part of their training. Unfortunately, young athletes may spend hours developing technical skills but neglect to develop good eating habits. There is a direct relationship between good sports nutrition and size, strength, endurance, conditioning, and injury prevention.

TIPS FOR HEALTHY EATING

Some youthful athletes believe they are paying attention to their diet when they consume expensive commercial dietary preparations, vitamins, amino acids, and other substances they believe will give them an edge on the playing field. The truth is that food works best. The three keys to choosing the best foods for healthful eating are as follows:

- Choose a variety of foods —don't eat the same diet every day.

- Eat sweets and fats in moderation.
- Balance proteins and fats into an overall carbohydrate-rich diet based on grains, fruits, and vegetables.

Weight is an important factor in performance of some sports, and it is common for athletes to severely restrict their diets in ways that ultimately harm their sports performance. Some athletes, like gymnasts and wrestlers, must be careful about gaining weight. One gymnast limited herself to plain yogurt, rice cakes, and oranges. Besides being boring, this diet also lacks iron, zinc, and vitamins A, E, and K. This is not a diet that supports high athletic performance, nor is it a wholesome diet.

To get wholesome food, choose natural or lightly processed foods. Select whole-wheat bread rather than white bread; choose a baked potato instead of potato chips. By opting for nutrient-dense foods, an athlete can get the recommended intake of most vitamins, minerals, and protein within a 1,200- to 1,500-calorie diet. Many active people do need to consume more calories (and thereby get more vitamins and minerals) on a daily basis. The number of calories depends on age, level of activity, body size, and gender.

A Time to Eat

Don't skip breakfast! Despite the fact that breakfast is undoubtedly the most important meal of the day, people in a hurry often omit it. "I don't have time." "I'm not hungry in the morning." "I don't like breakfast food." "If I eat breakfast, I feel hungrier all day." These are just a few of the familiar excuses. The truth is that skipping breakfast is a major nutritional mistake. A high-energy breakfast sets the tone for a high-energy day.

Breakfast need not be a sit-down, cooked meal to be nutritious. A banana and peanut butter sandwich works just fine for an athlete in a hurry. An early morning swimmer needs a healthful snack before practice—yogurt, a blender drink, bagel, or pita bread with a slice of low-fat cheese—and a full breakfast afterward. Exercised muscles are hungriest for carbohydrates within the first two hours after a workout.

Athletes who must control their weight should never skip breakfast. Research suggests that breakfast skippers struggle more with weight than breakfast eaters do. Breakfast calories are readily burned during a busy and active day. One study using individuals who

NUTRIENTS FOR HEALTH

Note: The U.S. Government has established recommended intakes to use as a guideline for dietary planning.

- Carbohydrate. Carbohydrates are the primary energy source during hard exercise, and they fuel muscle and the brain. About 60 percent of daily caloric intake (3 to 5 grams of carbohydrate per pound of body weight) should come from starches and carbohydrate-rich foods such as fruits, vegetables, breads, and grains.

- Fat. Fat is a source of stored energy that is burned primarily during low-level activity such as reading and sleeping. For good sports performance, limit fat intake to about 25 percent of daily total calories.

- Protein. Protein is an essential substance for building and repairing muscles, red blood cells, hair, and other tissues, and for synthesizing hormones. Protein can be used for energy when inadequate carbohydrate is available. About 15 percent of total daily calories should come from protein-rich foods such as fish, chicken, and dried beans.

- Vitamins. Vitamins are metabolic catalysts that regulate the chemical reactions within the body. Most are not manufactured by the body but are obtained through dietary selection. They are not a source of energy.

- Minerals. Minerals are elements obtained from foods that combine to form structures of the body (for example, calcium in bones). Important minerals are iron, magnesium, phosphorus, sodium, potassium, and zinc. They are not an energy source.

- Water. Water is an essential substance that makes up about 50 to 55 percent of body weight. Water stabilizes body temperatures, carries nutrients to cells, and carries waste products away from cells. It does not provide energy.

needed about 2,000 calories a day to maintain weight found that all the subjects lost weight when they ate their 2,000 calories at one morning meal. But when they moved the 2,000 calories to one evening meal, four of the six gained weight.

Snacking Right

Snack foods can be good for athletes who make wise food choices. Obviously, glazed donuts, Twinkies, M&Ms, chips, and pop provide fat and sugar, not healthful energy. On the other hand more healthful snacks such as dry cereal, popcorn, low-fat muffins, fruit, frozen fruit bars, crackers, bagels, baked potatoes, or nuts and seeds can boost energy and help maintain a better blood sugar level, which translates into sustained energy. An athlete who craves sweet snacks should look at whether overall calorie intake is adequate at meals and whether food intake has been delayed too long.

Eat Salads

Eat salads, but be careful with the dressing! Salad can be a nutrition bonus or a calorie-laden dietary disaster. A bowl of pale vegetables (iceberg lettuce, cucumber, celery) smothered in high-fat dressing offers little more than oil and crunch. Athletes can create a high-energy sports salad by selecting high-carbohydrate foods and limiting the fat. Veggies such as corn, peas, beets, and carrots are good sources of carbohydrates, as are beans and chick peas. Cooked rice, pasta, or potato chunks are other carbohydrate-dense ingredients. Choose low-fat or fat-free dressings, or dilute regular dressing with vinegar, lemon juice, or water. Don't add 800 to 1000 calories of regular fat-laden dressing. One bodybuilder gained weight on his so-called reducing diet because of his choice of salad dressing. At home, read labels and measure amounts.

Know Carbohydrates

Carbohydrates are the best choice for fueling muscles and promoting heart health. Carbohydrates should make up 60 percent of a healthful sports diet, and a wise athlete will study carbohydrates. Many athletes have misconceptions about this important dietary need that prevent them from making good carbohydrate choices.

Simple sugars are part of the carbohydrate family, including the monosaccharides (one-molecule sugars like glucose, fructose, and galactose) and the disaccharides (two-molecule sweeteners like sucrose or table sugar and milk sugar, which is a combination of glucose and galactose). Some athletes mistakenly believe that honey is nutritionally superior to refined white sugar, but it has no particular edge. Sugar in any form contains insignificant amounts of vitamins and minerals. A third type of sugar, known as glucose polymer, is a chain of about five glucose molecules that is the sweetener used in some of the popular sports drinks. Glucose polymer can provide more energy value with less sweetness than sugar.

In the body, all sugar and carbohydrates are digested into glucose before being burned as fuel. Both muscles and brain require blood glucose for energy and optimal brain function. Low blood sugar can cause an athlete to perform poorly because a poorly fueled brain limits muscular function and mental drive.

Complex carbohydrates (starches) are formed when sugars link together into long complex molecular chains. When starches are consumed, they are either burned for energy or stored for future use. Humans store extra dietary sugars in the form of muscle glycogen and liver glycogen, which is readily available for energy during exercise. Carbohydrate stores influence how long an athlete can exercise. When an individual runs low on glycogen, he or she feels overwhelmingly fatigued, a condition athletes call "hitting the wall."

The muscles mainly burn fat for energy when an individual is doing low-level exercise like typing. In light to moderate aerobic exercise, like jogging, stored fat provides 50 to 60 percent of the fuel. When an athlete exercises hard, like sprinting or weight lifting, energy comes primarily from glycogen stores. Moreover, biochemical changes that occur during exercise training influence the amount of glycogen that can be stored in muscle. Well-trained muscles can store two to three times more glycogen than untrained muscles, thus enhancing endurance.

To get energy, strength, and top sports performance, experts recommend the following:

- Eating carbohydrate-rich breakfasts like cereal rather than eggs.
- Focusing lunches and dinners on breads, potatoes, pasta, rice, fruits, and vegetables. At least two-thirds of the plate should be covered with these carbohydrates.
- Eating fish, chicken, lean meats, peanut butter, low-fat cheese, and other proteins as an accompaniment to meals, not as the main focus. At most, one-third of the dinner plate should be occupied by protein. Enjoy carbohydrate-rich protein alternatives such as beans and rice, lentil soup, chili, and other vegetarian choices.

These practices will ensure that athletes have carbohydrate, which is readily stored in muscles and available for exercise. One exercise physiologist compared the rate at which muscle glycogen was replaced in subjects who exercised to exhaustion and then ate either a high-protein/high-fat diet or a high-carbohydrate diet. Those on the high-protein/high-fat diet remained glycogen-depleted for five days. Subjects who ate the high-carbohydrate diet totally replenished muscle glycogen in two days. The conclusion: Carbohydrates are the better source of energy.

Athletes who train hard on a daily basis and need to maintain high energy will find carbohydrates a necessity. Glycogen depletion can occur if athletes don't take in enough carbohydrate while trying to maintain an exercise routine. In one study, athletes ran 10 miles on three consecutive days. They ate a diet that provided about 50 percent of calories from carbohydrates, which is less than the 60 to 65 percent that is recommended. The subjects found that their muscles became increasingly glycogen-depleted.

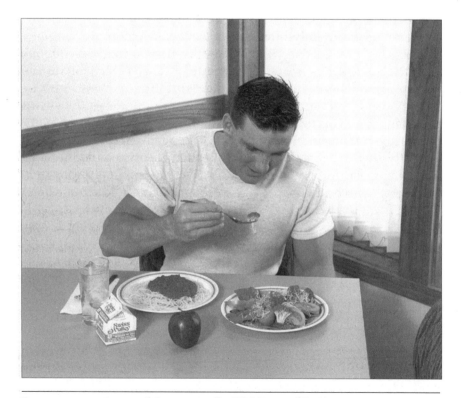

Boost energy and strength by eating a healthful mix of foods.

THE GOOD NUTRITION GAME PLAN

■ Dairy products. Best choices for dairy products are low-fat milk, yogurt, and low-fat cheese. Three or four daily servings of dairy products are needed for adequate calcium. Ice cream can be a fair source of calcium, but it contains excessive saturated fat and cholesterol. Try replacing it with frozen yogurt.

Remember that bones don't reach peak density until age 30 to 35. Adequate calcium helps maintain bone strength, protect against high blood pressure, protect against muscle cramps, and reduce the risk of osteoporosis in later life. Women who do not menstruate may need additional calcium.

■ Fruits and vegetables. Best choices in this group include oranges, bananas, melon, broccoli, spinach, green peppers, and tomatoes. The main nutrients are vitamins C and A, potassium, carbohydrates, fiber, and health-protective phytochemicals. These nutrients improve healing, reduce the risk of cancer, high blood pressure, and constipation, and aid recovery after exercise.

Eat at least two large (one cup) portions daily or four smaller portions. Bananas are a low-fat, high-fiber, high-potassium fruit that is perfect for busy athletes and even comes prewrapped! Orange juice fits nearly any diet and it has fewer calories and more nutrients than many other juices, including cranberry, apple, and grape. Because some vegetables have more nutritional value than many fruits, you can eat more veggies if eating fruit is a problem for you. Dark colorful vegetables have the most nutritional value, so select broccoli, spinach, green and red peppers, tomatoes, and carrots. Good sources of beta-carotene (for vitamin A) are carrots, winter squash, and greens.

■ Meats and protein-rich alternatives. Best choices in this category include lean meat, fish, poultry, nuts, beans, tofu, and legumes. Protein helps assure proper muscle development; the iron and zinc in animal protein reduces the risk of iron-deficiency anemia, and improves healing. Slabs of beef and huge hamburgers have no place in a sports diet, however. Extra protein isn't stored as muscle or muscle fuel.

Athletes can easily get too much protein in their diets. The recommended 4-ounce portion of meat is tiny compared to what most Americans eat: 12-ounce steaks, 8-ounce chicken breasts, 7-ounce cans of tuna. Because of its nutrients and lower fat content, a lean roast beef sandwich is preferable to grilled cheese, tuna salad, or a greasy hamburger. Poultry is relatively low in saturated fat. Fish may protect against heart disease and is a good source of protein. A few tablespoons of peanut butter are a convenient source of plant protein for vegetarians.

■ Grains and starches. Best choices in this category include whole-grain breads, cereals, and brown rice. The main nutrients are carbohydrates, fiber, and B vitamins. Protective benefits include fueling muscles, protecting against muscular fatigue, reducing problems with constipation, and being low in fat. The trick with eating carbohydrates is to avoid the fats that often accompany them—butter on bread, cream cheese on a bagel, oil on fried rice, and so on. This area is where many athletes fail in their quest for a low-fat, high-carbohydrate intake.

Some athletes eat too few carbohydrates because they think of them as fattening. Carbohydrates are not fattening. Fats are fattening, and many protein foods contain a lot of fat. Carbohydrates become fattening when they are covered with fats like butter, sour cream, mayonnaise, or greasy salad dressings or when the carbohydrates are eaten in excessive amounts.

Some athletes believe they are eating a high percentage of carbohydrates when they are not. One nutrition fanatic was stunned to find his diet was only 50 percent carbohydrates. Peanuts, almonds, granola, and sunflower seeds were adding fat to his diet. He traded them in for higher carbohydrate items like pretzels, raisins, dried apricots, and bananas and boosted his carbohydrate intake to 68 percent, with a resultant increase in athletic endurance.

A number of computer programs do dietary evaluation, which can be a valuable tool for individuals who want to control their diets. This service is not widely available at present, however. Check with hospitals, sports medicine clinics, or university medical centers for dietitians who do computerized dietary analysis.

Eating Fats

Although fats can be a major dietary pitfall for athletes, eliminating all fat from a sports diet is unwise. Nor should fats be eliminated without being replaced with adequate carbohydrates. A reasonable target for daily fat grams is 50 to 70 for women, and 60 to 90 grams of fat per day for men.

A LOOK AT SPORTS NUTRITION

Many athletes have questions about what to eat before, during, and after exercise.

Eating Before Exercise

Every athlete wants to know what to eat before exercising or competing. There is no one winning meal, and both physiological and psychological factors dictate the choice of pre-exercise food. However, any meal eaten before an event has four main functions:

- To help prevent hypoglycemia (low blood sugar), with its symptoms of light-headedness, fatigue, blurred vision, and indecisiveness, all of which can interfere with athletic performance
- To help settle the stomach, absorb gastric juices, and satisfy hunger feelings
- To fuel muscles, particularly in the case of food eaten far enough in advance to be digested and stored as glycogen
- To ease the mind with the knowledge that the body is well-fueled

From there, finding the right pretraining or precompetition meal is a matter of experimentation.

Carbo-Loading for Competition

To carbo-load for any athletic event that lasts for more than 90 minutes, an athlete should reduce the training regimen and rest muscles to allow them to become super-saturated with glycogen and consume a 60 to 70 percent carbohydrate diet for three days before the event.

Precompetition Dietary Guidelines

The following are some precompetition eating guidelines to help you maximize your sport performance:

- Eat high-carbohydrate meals daily for muscle fuel.

- Choose high-starch, low-fat foods that tend to digest easily, settle comfortably, and maintain stable blood sugar. Small servings of low-fat protein are permissible.

- Consume sugary foods with caution, especially within an hour of doing hard exercise. A "sugar boost" may cause a "sugar low" once exercise is begun. If you must have a sweet, eat it within 5 to 10 minutes of exercise because this is too short a time for the body to secrete excess insulin before exercise is begun and insulin secretion halts.

- Allow adequate time for food to digest. High-calorie meals take longer to leave the stomach than lighter snacks.

- Allow more digestion time before intense exercise (that you can sustain for 30 minutes) than before low-level activity. Muscles require more blood during intense exercise, and the stomach may get only 20 percent of its normal blood flow during a hard workout.

- Liquid foods leave the stomach faster than solids. Experiment to see whether liquid meals offer any advantages.

- Athletes who are jittery before competition should make a special effort to eat well the day before competition.

- Those who have a "magic food" should have it on hand. Even if you don't have a favorite food, you should have a snack on hand in case of delays.

- Always eat familiar foods before a competition; don't try out new foods.

- Drink plenty of fluids. Dehydration is possible with exercise so an athlete should drink an extra 4 to 8 glasses of fluid the day before competition and at least 2 or 3 glasses of water up to two hours before the event. Drink another 1 or 2 glasses up to 5 or 10 minutes before the start of the event.

Post-Exercise Nutrition

After an athlete has a hard workout, a top priority should be replacement of the fluids that were lost through sweating. Water is a conventional fluid. Juices supply water, carbohydrates, and electrolytes. Watery foods such as watermelon, grapes, and thin soups are also good. High-carbohydrate sports beverages or soft drinks supply fluids and carbohydrates but have few vitamins or minerals.

Within one to four hours after a workout, the athlete should consume carbohydrate-rich foods and more beverages. Extra protein beyond the recommended daily amount is not necessary. Minerals such as potassium can be replaced by eating fruits such as bananas or drinking juices. Replacing salt (sodium) loss is not a major concern for the average fitness participant as most meals contain adequate salt.

Drink Fluids

Drinking fluids cannot be overstressed. Many athletes who otherwise eat wisely neglect this essential step for top athletic performance. Thirst is not a guide to fluid needs. An athlete may not feel thirsty, but he or she still needs fluid. Body fluids play an important role in bodily function:

- Fluid in blood transports glucose to working muscles and carries away metabolic by-products.
- Fluid in urine eliminates metabolic waste products.
- Fluid in sweat dissipates heat through the skin.

When too little fluid is consumed or profuse sweating causes a heavy loss of fluid, it hinders the body's ability to accomplish these tasks, preventing the athlete from exercising at maximum potential. One way to judge whether fluid replacement is adequate is by the quantity and color of urine. Dark scanty urine is concentrated with metabolic wastes and is an indication that more water should be consumed. The body has returned to normal water balance when urine is clear or pale yellow.

Eight glasses of water a day is the suggested intake for adults, but that amount may not be enough for athletes. A general rule is to consume a liter of water (about one quart) for every 1,000 calories expended. Some athletes are concerned about drinking cold water, believing that it may cause stomach cramps. That is unlikely, and, in hot weather, drinking a cool fluid cools the body off faster. Drinking cool fluids in the winter, however, may be a poor choice for an athlete exercising outdoors in the cold.

Now that sports drinks have become popular, some athletes may believe that this type of beverage is necessary. Sports beverages are weak glucose solutions that can be quickly assimilated by the body during exercise. If a sports event lasts longer than 60 minutes, or is a short, intense, one-hour event, such as a soccer or hockey match, a beverage that contains a small amount of sugar can improve stamina. Sugar taken during exercise can enhance performance because the body does not secrete insulin during exercise. Plain water and carbohydrate snacks, such as hard candies, orange sections, or banana chunks are alternative choices for fluid and carbohydrates. An athlete should try different combinations to see what works best.

Protein and Performance

Traditional athlete fare has featured platefuls of beef, eggs, chicken, and other protein, with the premise that protein builds muscles. Extra protein does not build muscle bulk, however; strength training does that. Most athletes fall into two categories: the protein pushers (bodybuilders, weight lifters, football players) who think they can't get enough of it, and the protein avoiders (runners, triathletes, dancers) who never touch meat and who trade most protein calories for more carbohydrates. The truth is that dietary imbalances can cause both groups to perform poorly.

A small serving of protein-rich food at lunch and dinner should be adequate for the needs of healthy athletes. Vegetarians must be careful to get enough plant protein in their diets to maintain good health. One athlete lived on a diet of fruit for breakfast, a salad for lunch, and stir-fried vegetables with brown rice for dinner and believed she was eating healthy. She had the spindly arms and legs of an anorexic, however, and she had no menstrual periods, which is a sign of an unhealthy body. Also, a stress fracture healed very slowly, which is still another sign that her diet was inadequate for her exercise output.

Vitamin Supplements

Vitamin supplements are a big, almost unregulated business, and many claims are made that are excessive at the very least. Many athletes buy into the notion that they must supplement their diets with vitamins, protein powders, and amino acid pills. Some individuals may take a vitamin-pill breakfast to rationalize their chocolate chip cookie luncheons. Even if they get 100 percent of their vitamin needs with the breakfast pills, their bodies also need protein, minerals, energy, and fiber that they won't get with pills. Moreover, no scientific evidence proves that extra vitamins enhance performance, nor does exercising greatly increase vitamin needs.

Sometimes vitamin and mineral supplementation may be desirable:

- An inability to digest milk sugar may call for calcium supplementation.
- Expectant mothers and women hoping to become pregnant require additional vitamins and minerals.
- Total vegetarians may become deficient in vitamins B_{12}, D, and riboflavin.
- Dieters eating less than 1,200 calories daily may need supplementation.

Weight Control

Many athletes whose weight is perfectly normal are very concerned about gaining weight. It is almost a national obsession with many young women. Even among the nation's top women runners, a very lean group of women, weight is an issue. Excess body fat can slow an athlete down, but a certain amount of fat is needed for bodies to function well. Fat is an essential part of nerves, spinal cord, brain, and cell membranes.

Visual appearance and even body weight can be misleading because athletes compare themselves with their teammates. Bodies come in all sizes and shapes, however, and, for the most part, the size and shape is genetically determined. Athletes can change their bodies by losing or gaining weight, but they can't completely makeover their basic body type. Measuring the amount of body fat is a useful method for determining whether an athlete is at the correct weight. All methods of measuring body fat have the possibility of error, however, so body fat measurement should be used only as a guide to changes in the individual body.

Some athletes struggle to maintain proper weight levels, and some need to lose weight for top performance. High-energy, low-calorie reducing is possible, but it makes selecting the right foods more important. The body stores excess dietary fat as body fat very easily. Most dieters find that a high-carbohydrate/low-fat diet works better

TIPS FOR SUCCESSFUL DIETING

Follow these tips to meet your weight goals:

- Write down what you eat and drink in a day.
- Become aware of meal timing; consider consuming more calories earlier in the day.
- Roughly estimate the number of calories needed daily to maintain weight by multiplying present weight by 18 to 20 lb for moderately active athletes or by 23 to 25 lb for very active athletes. Subtract 20 percent from the maintenance number of calories needed to get the number of calories needed to reduce weight.
- Eat slowly. Overweight people tend to eat faster than normal-weight people. It takes 20 minutes for the brain to get the signal that enough nourishment has been consumed.
- Eat favorite foods on a regular basis. People who deny themselves foods they like are more likely to binge. When you eat the favorite food, chew slowly and savor the taste.
- Post a list of nonfood activities to do when bored, lonely, tired, or nervous.
- Use visualization to promote a positive attitude.

than a high-protein/low-carbohydrate diet and that they will also maintain a good energy level on this diet. The timing of meals also can enhance weight reduction. Dieters should eat mostly during the day so they have energy to exercise and reduce eating at night.

Weight Gain

Some athletes struggle to gain weight because they have inherited a genetic predisposition to thinness. Diet and weight training will help to some extent, but this type of athlete probably will not "bulk up." Consistently eating larger than normal meals and drinking extra fluids and lowfat milk are the best ways to gain weight. Also, having snacks at bedtime and eating high-calorie foods can help boost calorie intake.

Eating Disorders

Eating disorders among athletes seems to be on the rise, particularly in the weight-related sports such as gymnastics, running, wrestling, and lightweight crew. About a third of collegiate female athletes have some type of disordered eating pattern. Most food-obsessed athletes struggle on their own and are embarrassed that they cannot resolve their food imbalances. Athletes who are anorexic or bulimic are unlikely to be able to solve their food-related problems alone. They should seek help from a professional counselor experienced with eating disorders and nutritional guidance from a registered dietitian. Telephone the American Dietetic Association at 800-366-1655 for a referral to a nutritionist who has experience working with athletes who have eating disorders.

The Last Word

Eating for top exercise performance is becoming more scientific as we learn more about content of foods, timing of meals, and individual reactions to foods. Athletes who want advice on a particular aspect of eating should consult a registered dietitian in their area who specializes in working with athletes. Telephone the American Dietetic Association at 800-366-1655 for a referral.

Editor's Note: Nancy Clark is a Director of Nutrition Services at Boston-area's Sports Medicine Brookline. She has worked with many athletes to develop eating plans that enhance their sports activities. This chapter is adapted from her guide to good nutrition for athletes, *Nancy Clark's Sports Nutrition Guidebook,* Human Kinetics, 1997.

CHAPTER 11

TROUBLES WITH DRUG TESTING

Although drug testing is the primary method society has chosen to deal with the problem of college, professional, and Olympic athletes who choose to use banned substances, it is not a perfect method, and perhaps there never will be one. Nevertheless, as we look to the future, it is obvious that we cannot depend on drug testing alone to keep the playing field level.

We probably have always expected too much from drug testing, believing that policing athletic contests is all that is needed. Then, expecting too much, many of us are unreasonably disappointed when we find that drug testing is itself flawed. The magnitude of the crisis of confidence in drug testing was evident in the comments of Dr. Ralph Hale, vice president of the U.S. Olympic Committee (USOC), who said in an April 1995 interview published in the *New York Times*, "Our anti-doping campaign, I'm afraid, has been a failure to this point. Many countries have lost confidence in our anti-doping effort. I'm not sure we are doing the right job."

More harsh criticism of drug testing came in 1997 from an article in *Sports Illustrated*. After a lengthy investigation of drug use at the elite level, the authors of the article concluded that "drug testing is serving as no deterrent" (page 70). According to the article, "Dozens of athletes, coaches, administrators, and steroid traffickers interviewed by *SI* say that the Atlanta Olympics, like other Games of the last half century, was a carnival of sub-rosa experiments in the use of performance-enhancing drugs. A few of those interviewed were surprised that only two users were caught" (page 62).

These are strong words. Certainly, others believe that drug testing has worked about as well as it could. Looking at the scorecard for drug testing to date, Don Catlin, MD, head of the first IOC-accredited drug testing laboratory in the United States, says, "We've been successful in a couple of areas. We knocked out all the short-acting drugs such as amphetamines, beta blockers, and other drugs that must be taken at the time of competition. We obviously pushed the casual anabolic steroid user out, the person who was really just experimenting on his own. But we are left with a base of hard-core users who understand exactly what laboratories can and can't do and who try to evade testing. It's a big issue."

Dr. Catlin is director of the Olympic Analytical Facility at the University of California at Los Angeles and a member of the IOC Medical Commission. He is a realist, as is John Baenziger, MD, director of clinical pathology at the Indiana University Medical Center in Indianapolis, home of the other IOC-accredited drug testing laboratory in the United States. "Drug testing cannot stand on its own as a deterrent," Dr. Baenziger says flatly. "It's just a tool, a sampling technique that lets us see what is going on. The laboratory cannot do everything." Both laboratory directors agree that unless the sports-governing bodies, the athletes themselves, and the public demand clean competition and an end to chemical cheating, the testing laboratories often find themselves fighting a rear guard action.

The major problems with drug testing are as follows:

■ Some athletes who cheat are not caught.
■ The secrecy that surrounds all testing makes it difficult for athletes to believe their interests are being protected and for the public to understand what is going on.
■ Sports-governing bodies control nearly every aspect of the testing process.
■ Political maneuvering, both within the IOC itself and among nations, causes problems.

ATHLETES WHO CHEAT

Much as we might wish it weren't true, athletes are getting away with using banned performance-enhancing drugs. When drug use goes undetected, athletes may achieve personal success, but the overall impact on sports is negative. Suspecting a competitor of using drugs is extremely discouraging and frustrating to those athletes who have made many personal sacrifices to continue competing in their sports without drugs.

There have been instances where the circumstances surrounding an athlete's performance make it highly likely that drug use is occurring. However, without confirmation by drug testing, nothing can be done. For instance, it strains credulity to see swimmers nearly 10 years older than the rest of the field improve times as they get older. When links to previous drug use or with known drug users exist, it becomes even harder to believe that success is not drug-aided.

Passing a drug test does not mean that a particular athlete does not use drugs. Canadian sprinter Ben Johnson successfully passed 19 drug tests in the two years before he was caught by a drug test at the 1988 Olympic Games in Seoul. At the Canadian hearings, he admitted to long-standing use of steroids, which means he had negative drug tests at a time when he was using the drugs to aid his performance. The false negatives are "much higher than we should have," Dr. Catlin acknowledges.

Moreover, there have been cases where there was, in his words, clearly "an intent to dope" on the part of the athlete, as opposed to a simple mistake. For instance, there were many positive tests for bromantan at the 1996 Games in Atlanta. In a controversial decision, the International Court of Arbitration for Sport ruled that these should not be considered positive drug tests because the IOC did not provide sufficient evidence that bromatan is a performance-enhancing drug, but the fact remains that bromantan is a drug, and it is not a substance that athletes would take in a normal training regimen, unless they were looking for performance enhancement.

Lack of Tests

Another factor contributing to athletes not getting caught is a lack of effective tests for certain drugs. At present, there is no test to detect the presence of human growth hormone (hGH), which is used by power and strength athletes for its anabolic (muscle-building) effects. According to the *Sports Illustrated* article cited earlier, some athletes jokingly referred to the Atlanta Olympics as the "Growth Hormone Games" (page 66). A related anabolic hormone, insulin-like growth factor (IGF-1), is also available to athletes, and it too has no effective test. There is also no test as yet for erythropoietin (EPO), which is used by endurance athletes to increase the number of red blood cells and thus improve their oxygen-carrying capacity.

There is little doubt that these three very powerful drugs help athletic performance, and there are other hormones in this class of banned substances that athletes use to enhance athletic performance as well. Dr. Catlin says that some progress is being made, particularly for human chorionic gonadotropin. Also, in 1996, the IOC, in partnership with a consortium of European academic centers and pharmaceutical companies, began a 2 million dollar program to develop a test for human growth hormone by the Olympic Games of 2000 in Sydney. Others argue that 2 million dollars represents less than a sincere effort on the part of a billion-dollar business, the IOC, to deal with the most serious problem threatening sports today. Clearly, the research and development expenditures of a comparable size pharmaceutical company would dwarf the IOC's investment.

Significant numbers of Olympic athletes have probably used creatine, a substance found naturally in the body that has been demonstrated to enhance performance. It does not appear on the banned list because it supposedly is a food supplement. However, a person would need to eat more than 10 to 20 pounds of meat a day to equal the standard loading dose now being taken by athletes: easy for a tiger, tough for a human!

The Trouble With the T/E Ratio

Another problem affecting testing is the fact that far too much latitude exists in the T/E ratio. Testosterone, the main male sex hormone, occurs naturally in the bodies of both men and women, and conventional gas chromatography/mass spectrometer testing cannot distinguish between testosterone that was produced in the body and testosterone taken in from outside. That may be about to change in the near future, given that Dr. Catlin has developed a test that may distinguish between natural and synthetic testosterone. But until that test becomes a reality, drug testing still has a major problem with testosterone.

In another signal of concern about testosterone, the USOC appointed a blue-ribbon panel to investigate the issue and make recommendations for improving testing procedures and systems. Because this panel was announced just one month after Dr. Catlin's testosterone test was reported, some observers were concerned about the timing. If a foolproof test for testosterone is now available, why would the USOC even consider removing testosterone from the list of banned drugs? Whether the concern is valid, in the absence of a definitive test it is certain that drug testing will continue to be plagued with the problem of testosterone.

In deciding how much testosterone is too much, drug testers use a ratio of testosterone to epitestosterone, another naturally occurring hormone. Most normal men have a ratio of about $1/1$, but the distribution of this ratio by race, age, body fat, hydration status, diet, and level of conditioning has not been well-established in the peer-reviewed medical literature. Even less information is available on

THE TESTOSTERONE PROBLEM

The critical and controversial issue of testosterone use will be considered by a panel of medical experts assembled by the United States Olympic Committee. Members of the panel include:

- Dr. Donald I. Macdonald, founder and chairman/CEO of Employee Health Programs, Inc.
- Dr. Ronald S. Swerdloff, professor of medicine at UCLA and chief of the Division of Endocrinology and Metabolism at Harbor-UCLA Medical Center
- Dr. William J. Bremner, professor and vice-chairman of the Department of Medicine at the University of Washington
- Dr. Richard V. Clark, research and development specialist with Glaxo Wellcome and former professor at Emory and Duke

The directors of the IOC-accredited laboratories in the United States will serve as nonvoting advisory members. They are Dr. Catlin of UCLA and Dr. Larry Bowers of the Sports Medicine and Drug ID Laboratory at Indiana University.

women, although it does appears that women's rates fluctuate more than men's do and are probably affected by monthly hormonal changes.

To avoid false accusations, the IOC set the ratio at 6/1. Unfortunately, athletes can take enough testosterone to help them with their sports performance before they reach the 6/1 level. That is especially true for women athletes. Even a small amount of testosterone may be enough for them to make substantial improvements. According to Dr. Catlin, athletes who use testosterone in this way do sometimes slip and go over the limit, more often than might be imagined. Given the availability of relatively new ways of slowly releasing testosterone into the body through skin patches and gels, however, these slips are likely to be less frequent.

In addition to these problems, there may well be designer drugs and masking agents created by chemists working for the drug-using factions that are as yet unknown. Although the IOC-approved laboratories in this country are without peer, they can only find that for which they can test.

Over-the-Counter Drugs

Another problem connected to drug testing is the fact that the IOC regulations on over-the-counter (OTC) drugs, such as cold medications, cough syrup, asthma medications, and even headache pills, are often unclear and confusing. Even though hundreds of OTC drugs are banned, the IOC permits the use of at least that many. Most doctors believe the list is too long and that it can, in fact, interfere in the proper medical treatment of athlete patients.

Dr. Gary Wadler, a New York internist and senior author of the book *Drugs and the Athlete*, has pointed out that there is little evidence that most of these OTC remedies enhance sports performance, even in larger doses than an athlete would take to treat a medical condition. The IOC does not specify how much of an OTC drug is too much, however. Wadler also contends that some elite athletes overreact to mild stimulants such as those found in many cold medications, causing greater than normal amounts of the metabolic by-products to be present in their urine. This difference may lead testers to believe a drug has been abused when it was taken at a normal dosage.

The lack of clear direction has caused some athletes to avoid treatment for minor illnesses, such as colds or sinus infection. Under the IOC rules, however, athletes are permitted to take nonsteroidal painkillers even though taking away pain can certainly improve sports performance. Thus, an athlete may compete with an untreated cold, but he can take medication for pain.

Some drugs used to treat asthma are in the prohibited class known as β_2 agonists. Some drugs in this class have been used by athletes purportedly for their anabolic (tissue building) effects, their fat burning effects, as well as their muscle sparing effects during dieting and intense exercise. Three drugs in this class (terbutaline, salbutamol, and salmeterol) can be used if they are administered by inhalation, and if their use is declared in advance on a special form. By permitting only the inhaled form, the Medical Commission thought it unlikely that enough could be taken to enhance performance.

A request to use these drugs or the inhaled corticosteroids that are commonly given to treat asthma must be submitted in writing by the Olympic team physician of each country. In an article in the *Journal of the American Medical Association*, Dr. Catlin disclosed that in some sports, more declarations were submitted than could be accounted for by the normal incidence of asthma in the standard population. This fact leads to the speculation that a significant number of athletes may be trying to use these drugs for performance enhancement, regardless of whether they work.

SECRECY IN THE LABORATORY

There are strong arguments for maintaining a curtain of secrecy around the sports drug-testing process. Secrecy is intended to protect the athlete's right to privacy and the integrity of the drug-testing process. Who has a right to drug-testing information is a sensitive matter. Many believe this information is private, to be shared only with the athlete and the appropriate sports-governing bodies; others believe the public should be informed.

Many people in sports, both athletes and administrators, subscribe to the view that the public has no right to know about the drug habits of any athlete. They also point out that not every positive test represents an attempt to cheat. The IOC list of banned drugs is quite lengthy, and anabolic steroids are only a part of it. As noted, an athlete could get a positive test by taking a certain type of cold medication. Should that athlete be branded as a cheat? There are both legal and ethical dimensions to the situation.

Then there is the matter of secrecy relative to the drug testing procedure itself. Most reputable people in drug testing do not want to share their cutting-edge technology with just anyone. They note, quite correctly, that drug users also read and would be all too happy to know exactly what can and cannot be done in the laboratory. This information could then be used in a way that would harm athletes and sports competition in general. On the other hand, some have argued that the testers are not held to the same scientific standards as other medical scientists in that they often have been slow to publish the details and accuracy standards of their various tests in peer-reviewed professional journals.

How can the public be sure that drug testing is carried out in a fair and impartial manner and that the process is relatively free of error? Secrecy could serve to cover up errors or inconsistencies in the testing process if they occur. The concern over this aspect of the secrecy surrounding testing is legitimate in that the reputation and livelihood of athletes are clearly at stake. Nevertheless, it takes a great deal of time and effort to maintain state-of-the-art knowledge in such a sophisticated drug market, and laboratories don't want to share their knowledge with individuals who would use it for personal benefit.

To what extent variations in economic resources and political goals has affected the incidence of false positive or false negative tests has never been publicly documented. Relatively well funded operations like Dr. Catlin's lab at UCLA or Dr. Baenziger's lab in Indianapolis have more resources and likely do higher quality work.

Dr. Baenziger observed that the two IOC-accredited U.S. laboratories are the only two in the entire 25-institution IOC network that routinely go through published proficiency testing. This does not mean, he notes, that they are the only ones doing excellent work, just that it is hard to compare laboratories in different countries. Dr. Baenziger notes that the laboratory personnel must not only keep up with abused drugs, but must also be on the lookout for new ones and for agents that mask the presence of banned substances. Dr. Craig Kammerer, senior scientist at Arimenterics, Inc., observes that there is a great deal of interest currently in the natural compounds, the hormones and polypeptides. Because these substances are found naturally in the body, it will be difficult to demonstrate what quantity came from outside the body; in fact, such information does not exist presently. One newcomer on the performance-enhancing scene is orotic acid, a sort of vitamin that Dr. Kammerer says athletes use because it has both anabolic properties and the potential to mask the presence of other drugs.

All these issues come down to the two important questions that have not, as yet, been answered to the satisfaction of all:

- Can drug use be curtailed or eliminated within a secret system?
- Does the public have any right to drug testing results?

Even when great care is taken in handling the specimens and in doing the actual laboratory work, the economic and political conditions in various countries affect the operations of drug testing laboratories. Not all laboratories are equal, either in expertise in testing nor in political position. Some countries still view athletics as an extension of national image, and they take a keen interest in seeing their athletes succeed.

We now know that scientists at the government's IOC-approved DKL laboratory in the former East Germany played a major role in helping East German athletes circumvent drug tests. Government documents recovered after the fall of East Germany revealed that the laboratories kept track of washout times for steroids and experimented with dosage levels of testosterone to bridge the times when athletes would be off other steroids.

THE JESSICA FOSCHI CASE

A case that illustrates some of the potential problems with drug testing is that of Jessica Foschi, now 17, an Olympic hopeful in swimming. She tested positive for the anabolic steroid mesterolone, not legally available in North America, at the U.S. Swimming national championships in 1995, which normally would result in a two-year ban from competition. However, in October 1995, a review board of U.S. Swimming voted 2-1 to place her on probation for two years. Members of the review board, which included two former Olympic swimmers, said they were convinced that Foschi was the victim of sabotage and cited the unusually high amount of the steroid present when she was tested.

Foschi and her parents did not question the drug test itself, which was performed at the IOC-approved laboratory at UCLA. The results of that test revealed one of the highest levels of mesterolone ever seen in a male or female athlete. However, the family and coach continued to insist they had nothing to do with steroids, and all passed lie detector tests administered by internationally recognized experts. A medical examination showed that it was very improbable that Foschi was a chronic steroid user, and follow-up drug tests were all negative.

If Foschi was the victim of sabotage, it marks the first known case in U.S. sports. Several experts who have been consulted on this case indicated they agreed with the review board members who concluded that this was sabotage. However, this case put U.S. Swimming in an embarrassing position in that it has been critical of Chinese swimmers who tested positive for anabolic steroids. A number of U.S. Swimming administrators, including President Carol Zaleski, said that although they believe that Foschi did not intentionally take a banned substance, intent is irrelevant, and Foschi should be banned. This stance is based on the premise that the athlete must be on guard against sabotage.

The case took another strange turn when FINA, the international sports governing body for swimming, acted favorably on the case of an Australian swimmer who had taken a non-steroid banned substance. At that point, U.S. Swimming reversed its position and ruled that Foschi could swim without sanctions, but placed her on probation for two years. Thereafter, the American Arbitration Association also found in favor of Jessica, reaffirmed her innocence, and overturned the probation. Meanwhile, the Foschi family brought suit against U.S. Swimming and the USOC, an action that was settled out of court when U.S. Swimming agreed to pay $92,000 toward Jessica's legal expenses. She competed in the Olympic Trials for swimming in March 1996, but she did not make the team. Since that time, FINA reviewed the Foschi case and suspended her for a two-year period. The case then went before the International Court of Arbitration for Sport, which reversed FINA's ruling, reduced the suspension to six months (which Jessica had already served), and ordered FINA to pay approximately $10,000 toward Jessica's legal expenses. Meanwhile, in the summer of 1996, Jessica won the national 5K open water championship in Ft. Lauderdale, Florida, swimming 3.1 miles in 1 hour, 14 minutes, and 33 seconds, in only her second open water swim.

One other U.S. woman swimmer, Angel Martino Martin, had a positive test for steroids, and she was removed from the Olympic team competing in Seoul in 1988. Martin came back from her two-year suspension and competed for the United States in Barcelona and again in Atlanta, where she won three medals while competing as one of the oldest female swimmers in the pool. She contends her previous positive test was a mistake.

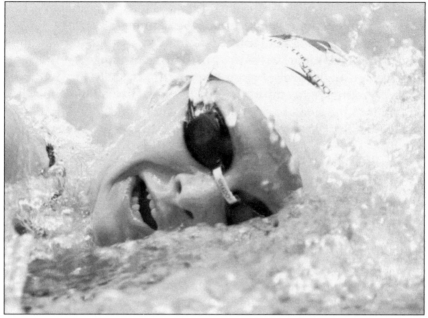

Jessica Foschi is one of many athletes who have tested positive for steroids and claimed the results were sabotaged or faulty due to poor testing procedures.

CONTROL BY SPORTS-GOVERNING BODIES

The present case wherein the sports-governing bodies are also the ones to control testing is complicated. Who has a stronger interest in promoting sports than the sports-governing bodies? Who will be more harmed than the sports-governing bodies when there is a public perception of widespread drug use? This potential stumbling block in the drug-testing procedure is well-recognized. As Dr. Catlin has said, "As long as sport is charged with being both the promoter of athletes and the punishers, there is an inherent conflict of interest."

Robert Voy, MD, former director of sports medicine for the USOC, has been very outspoken about the situation. In his book, *Drugs, Sport, and Politics*, he commented, "Allowing national governing bodies, international federations, and national Olympic Committees, such as the United States Olympic Committee, to govern the testing process to ensure fair play in sport is terribly ineffective. In a sense, it is like having the fox guard the henhouse."

Obviously, no sports organization, amateur or professional, wants to see its athletes identified as drug users. A clean image is important. A perceived high level of drug use could adversely impact ticket sales, TV ratings, and endorsements. To a great extent, the public has bought into the clean image of athletes, and it doesn't want to hear that the feats of its favorite sports heroes may have been steroid-aided.

Public reaction to steroid use is one of the most interesting aspects of the problem. At least some segments of the public have decided, in some subtle way, that steroid use among elite athletes is not a matter of genuine public health concern because these athletes are viewed as mercenaries or entertainers who take calculated risks in return for large amounts of money. This view persists despite the fact that these drugs expose users to health risks, render any athletic contest unfair, and tacitly endorse the concept of cheating to gain an advantage. Moreover, a drug testing system, particularly one that doesn't work very well, allows sports federations plausible deniability while continuing to provide the fan with superhuman athletes performing record-breaking feats.

The sports-governing bodies act in what they believe to be the best interests of their individual sport when they make their drug policies. Although it would be wrong to assume that the sports-governing bodies are not motivated by love of the sport and a wish to serve and protect their athletes, the fact is that they also must be aware of their major financial interest and guard their public image. They recognize that the public does not want to perceive athletes as drug users.

Different sports-governing bodies approach the issue of doping control differently. Some have extensive programs, both in-competition and short-notice. Others have only the most minimal effort. According to Dr. Catlin, the number of positive cases correlates with the sophistication and quality of the doping control program. He believes that most of the severely affected sports have responded by increasing doping funding and by making genuine efforts to curtail the problem. How this sense of optimism is affected by the recent decision of the International Amateur Athletics Federation (IAAF, the international governing body for track and field) to reduce the suspension penalty for a first-time steroid offense from four years to two is unclear.

In the spring of 1995, USA Track & Field stopped collecting urine samples until it could put a new program in place that would be more of a deterrent. Under their short-notice testing system, athletes had 48 hours to produce a sample, which gave them time to beat the tests, as demonstrated by the fact that the program had not produced a positive result since 1991. Their plan now is to adopt a no-notice immediate testing plan. The complexity of the hearing process of USA Track & Field kept runner Mary Decker Slaney in competition after a positive test for testosterone.

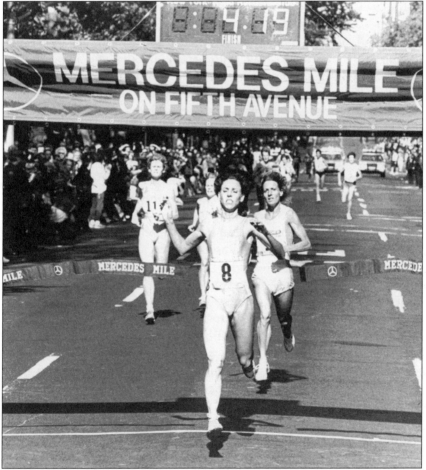

©UPI/Corbis-Bettmann

Mary Decker Slaney exceeded the allowed limit for testosterone and was banned from competition temporarily until track and field governing bodies conceded the possibility of a false positive.

Eight national NGBs in high risk sports are now participating in a pilot program for out-of-competition testing. USOC Vice President Ralph Hale sees this participation as a promising avenue of action. "We felt it was time to bring (drug testing) back as a major issue," he said. "We've got to get people's attention." This new no-notice testing program will still not be able to detect hGH, IGF-1, or EPO, however. Nor is it likely to catch many athletes who use testosterone through skin gels or patches.

The National Football League was rocked by unfavorable publicity during the 1970s and 1980s as details of widespread use of steroids in the NFL emerged. Even though most knowledgeable observers say steroid use continues at a high level in football, the sport has successfully distanced itself from association with drugs by changing the way it handles testing. The current NFL drug testing program policy of treating steroid use as a private matter invokes the curtain of secrecy first described by journalist Jim Ferstle. Now it is impossible to know whether progress has been made.

Linemen are definitely much larger than they were 20 years ago. A professional football player remarked recently that when two of these massive bodies slam together at speed on the field, the physical damage is greater than it used to be. Players compete with pain more often, and injuries are up. Some current professional football players say steroid use has declined sharply in the NFL, but retired players often just smile at that notion. In truth, there is no way to know.

Jerry Jones, owner of the Dallas Cowboys, suggested in a newspaper interview that each team should handle all drug issues for its players, saying that nobody else would have more interest in the well-being of the players. In a sport where alcohol abuse has been widespread for many years and tacitly accepted by most teams, how likely is it that football owners will be concerned if they have bigger, stronger players?

The fact that many sports organizations have deliberately gone very low-profile on steroid testing has convinced a large segment of the public that steroids were a fad that swept the country and faded, like love beads and bell-bottom jeans. This belief flies in the face of strong evidence that says the level of drug use is about what it has always been. Moreover, the use of testosterone patches and gels appears to have increased greatly in sports like major league baseball almost without any public notice.

Olympians Pat and Harold Connolly have spent years speaking

out against widespread steroid use in track and field. Pat Connolly now sums up the situation this way, "Just writing a rule hasn't stopped it. Instead of spending money on testing, we need to spend money on research. After a lifetime of argument and debate on the subject (of drug testing), there is not much more you can do."

THE POLITICS OF DRUG TESTING

Another politically charged issue in drug testing is how positive tests are handled. Some athletes and coaches have expressed the belief that athletes have been framed in the past. Whether this belief has any merit, it exists and creates divisiveness between testers and athletes. Dr. Catlin has noted that the subject of sabotage is complex because it can never be excluded and rarely can be proved.

The IOC itself has been stung by charges it deliberately withheld the names of athletes with positive tests for political reasons. Obviously, detecting a large number of drug-using athletes would harm the public image of the Olympic Games. Because the IOC is generally accountable only to itself, it is hard to know where the truth lies. We know, for instance, that at the 1980 Olympic Games in Moscow (the United States did not send a team), there were no positive tests. After the Games were over, however, Professor Manfred Donike, one of the most influential figures in drug testing, took urine samples back to his laboratory in Cologne, Germany (as he had always done), and found striking evidence of widespread use of testosterone. Testosterone was not specifically banned at the time, although its use violated the spirit of the rules.

Certainly, there have been rumors since 1988 that there was an attempt to suppress the positive test of Canadian sprinter Ben Johnson. This rumor was fueled by the fact that there apparently was a leak that resulted in the news media hearing about the positive test before it was officially announced.

Something definitely happened in 1984 at the Summer Games in Los Angeles as well. Although a formal cover-up of positive tests has been alleged, even now, more than a decade later, nobody is sure what took place or who was responsible. In brief, a scientific paper published by Dr. Catlin and his associates after the Games showed significant discrepancies with the official count of positive tests. Dr. Catlin, who was not a member of the IOC Medical Commission at the time, says, "I knew the day after the Games when I wasn't ordered to test some of the B samples that there was a discrepancy. We all knew about it and were very concerned about it."

Dr. Catlin's lab at UCLA tested 1,510 samples that came to the laboratory during the 1984 Games and were identified only by code numbers. As is always the case, the master list that pairs code and athlete name was held by Prince De Merode in his capacity as head of the Medical Commission. Several parties, including Dr. Arnold Beckett, former head of the IOC-approved drug testing laboratory in London and a founding member of the Medical Commission, suspect that someone in the IOC deliberately covered up positive tests.

Prince De Merode's explanation for the situation in 1984 has been that there was a burglary at his hotel. At the end of the Games, he opened the locked cabinet that had contained the master list and found it gone. Neither he nor the other members of the Medical Commission, Dr. Donike, Dr. Beckett, and Dr. Robert Dugall, then head of the IOC-approved drug laboratory in Montreal, knew how the code list disappeared, and it has remained a mystery. In his book, *The New Lords of the Rings*, journalist Andrew Jennings reported that the cabinet was forced open and the documents removed and shredded, although it still is unknown who gave the order.

Now it appears that the "lost tests" from Atlanta may raise suspicions again about high-level suppression of positive tests. Several months after the 1996 Olympic Games in Atlanta, it was revealed that somewhere between two and five positive tests were not reported. When this fact finally became known, the official explanation given was that some test results had unfortunately been lost but that it probably was not as many as five. Bear in mind, also, that none of the "lost tests" were those that were positive for bromantan.

Losing test results casts no reflection on the heads of the drug-testing laboratories who never, in any case, have in their possession, the master list that pairs the number on a urine sample with the name of a particular athlete. That list is held by one man, Prince De Merode, and he is accountable to Juan Antonio Samaranch, head of the International Olympic Committee.

We live in a time when many people believe in conspiracies, sometimes on the flimsiest of evidence. When we consider how the Ben Johnson episode from the 1988 Games in Seoul cast such a long shadow over sports, it becomes less difficult to imagine that if there were a positive test for a top athlete at a Games that already had undergone many rocky moments, there might be strong sentiment for the test to simply disappear. For the protection of the top officials of the IOC, it might be better to devise another way of pairing the codes and reporting results so that those suspicions could not arise.

Dr. Catlin has already said he hopes that moving to a system whereby laboratories report simultaneously to the IOC and the international sports-governing bodies will circumvent some of the problems now inherent in the system. He says he is very supportive of an open system where everything is reported all around. If simultaneous reports are made to more than one body, it would be more difficult to suppress positive results.

He also noted that many people assume that the purpose of drug testing is to protect athletes from harming themselves. In his view, the primary reason has more to do with the meaning of sports, and he says that the rules of sport "create a structure in which athletes compete to display manifestations of human·excellence that are prized and admired." In that sense, drug testing is an effort to preserve what is beautiful in sports and to make the playing field level for all.

Dr. Baenziger says, "I do feel that drug testing is a deterrent and that is has an impact on the amount of use. So for that purpose only, I think it's still effective. Whether drug testing can eliminate drug use...well, I'm not that optimistic. There will always be the potential for people to cheat." Both directors note that as long as money and fame drive international sports, athletes have a very strong incentive to use whatever leverage they can obtain.

COMMENTS BY DR. Y

I would argue that the sole reason for drug testing is to protect the image of the Olympics, the NFL, and other sport federations as defenders of the noble and pure pursuit of athletic excellence. The commercialization of sport is obvious—it is now a multibillion dollar business, and the cheating and subversive nature inherent in illicit drug use is very bad for business. If the fans believed that drug use was pervasive in the Olympics and professional sport, would they have flocked to Atlanta by the thousands and paid exorbitant prices for tickets, hotel rooms, and meals? Would millions of Americans sit glued to their television each Sunday watching football? Some would still watch, but many would not, and the sport business would suffer. Enter drug testing.

The IOC contracts with highly competent and reputable scientists who use the most sophisticated equipment to do drug testing. The IOC has a mantra which then is recited, "While drug use has been a problem in the past, we now have these new tests and this new equipment. Problem solved." There is nothing wrong with the IOC mantra per se except that, like all mantras, it is repeated over and over while few question its accuracy. I heard it in the 1970s, the 1980s, and now again in the 1990s.

In 1972, the U.S. Senate held hearings that documented widespread steroid use in sport, including the Olympics. The IOC countered by introducing in-competition testing for steroids at the 1976 Montreal Games. Problem solved. The IOC proved its point by referring to the fact that less than two percent of the thousands of athletes that participated in the 1976, 1980, and 1984 Olympics Games tested positive for performance-enhancing drugs. In the 1980 Games, no one tested positive!

In 1988 when Ben Johnson tested positive for steroids, some people asked how he was able to pass his previous 19 drug tests. The IOC was forced to publicly acknowledge a problem with in-competition testing that it had known about since the inception of testing for steroids in 1976; such testing only worked on those few athletes who were careless and did not discontinue their use in time for the drug to clear their body. The IOC quickly offered a solution: short-notice (48 hours), out-of-competition testing. Problem solved.

In the 1990s, when rumors of drug use of epidemic proportions persisted even with short-notice testing, Dr. Ralph Hale, vice-president of the U.S. Olympic Committee, acknowledged the failure of the drug-testing program but immediately offered yet another solution in the form of newer and even more sophisticated equipment as well as requiring no-notice testing. Once again the problem is solved, and the fans are reassured.

This public relations strategy is starting to come unglued due in part to the efforts of journalists who have started to bring to the public domain knowledge that was previously reserved for a small number of scientists and most sport federation officials. For example, testosterone can be applied with skin gels or patches such that detection is highly unlikely, especially among women. Other examples are that there are no tests for human growth hormone, IGF-1, and erythropoietin. But fear not, the IOC has promised that this problem will be solved by the 2000 Games in Sydney.

Because testing is fraught with so many loopholes, we still don't know how many Olympic athletes or NFL players are using performance-enhancing drugs. In the mid 1980s, unannounced drug tests with no punitive actions were conducted at a U.S. national track and field meet. Fifty percent of the athletes tested positive! Are today's athletes more ethical than those of a decade past? I am skeptical. I also feel sorry for the innocent athletes who have to suffer that skepticism.

Both my coauthor and I have strongly held opinions about drug testing, although our perspectives differ slightly. Here is what she says about this important issue:

"In my opinion, drug testing is a reasonable effort to stem the use of performance-enhancing drugs, and progress has been made. It would be a step in the wrong direction to weaken the drug testing effort. If we were left without that line of defense, many athletes would be forced to make the unpalatable choice of competing unsuccessfully in their sports or taking drugs. The war on recreational drugs in this country waxes and wanes, but that does not mean it should be abandoned. So it is with performance-enhancing drugs.

The discrepancies in test results from Atlanta, however, are deeply disturbing. Working as a volunteer at one of the venues,

I saw firsthand the effort expended by so many people who believe in and admire the Olympic movement in its purer form. I am convinced that there were medalists in Atlanta who cheated with drugs and were not caught, but it would be painful to learn that positive tests were deliberately suppressed. If drug testing is to succeed, it must be fairly administered and fairly reported. We cannot accept drug use as part of the normal course of events."

CHAPTER 12

PREPARING FOR THE FUTURE

Looking to the future, it is easy to identify the hazards that performance-enhancing drugs bring to sport, but it is hard to agree on an appropriate course of action and follow it. In addition to steroid abuse, athletes also are using human growth hormone, insulin-like growth factor, erythropoietin, and a myriad of other drugs. As researchers continue to unlock the chemical secrets of the human body, it is reasonable to assume that additional drugs that confer an athletic advantage will be developed. If Americans cannot agree on how to deal with the drugs we have now, there can be no basis for deciding how to handle future drugs that may be used to alter physiology or psychology.

This problem is not new. Cheating was known even in the original Olympic games in ancient Greece. In the modern world, man's capacity to alter body and mind brings a new dimension to an old problem. At the 1993 Prague Conference on Steroids, delegates agreed on a series of reasons why performance enhancement in sports is unacceptable, including the following:

- An athlete may suffer physical or psychological harm because of his drug use.

- Drug use contaminates sport because the results are obtained by unnatural means. An athlete who uses drugs has an unfair advantage over one who does not.
- The use of anabolic steroids is cheating and violates the rules of virtually every sport.
- The use of steroids for nonmedical purposes is a violation of state and federal laws.
- The use of drugs by one athlete may coerce or force another to use them to maintain equality.
- High school students and younger individuals are using these drugs.

If the only thing wrong with steroids were a risk to health, an athlete would be justified in taking a position that it is a matter of individual choice whether to accept that risk. However, these drugs have the power to fundamentally change the contest because they change the strength and power of the contestants. Therefore, the ethical and moral must be addressed.

A FOCUS ON WINNING

The fact is that the appetite for steroids and other performance-enhancing drugs has been created predominantly by a societal fixation on winning and physical appearance. This behavior is learned. Children play games for fun, at least as long as they can before adults intervene to tell them that winning is what's important. One of the strongest reasons we should not give up the struggle to

THE WRONG MESSAGE

A 10-year-old suburban Chicago youngster got a hands-on lesson in looking for an edge in 1995. Players in his private youth football league are divided by weight, under or over 85 pounds. Kids who are big for their age have to play with older athletes, and most don't like to do this because they lack the necessary skills to play successfully. According to the front-page article in the September 1, 1995 issue of *The Chicago Tribune,* the youth took a strong prescription diuretic drug, Lasix, to lose weight quickly so he could make the lower weight classification. Lasix is sometimes used by horse owners to cause heavy urination in their horses to reduce their race weight. The child, who normally weighs about 94 pounds, lost about 10 percent of his body weight over a period of several hours. At the weigh-in, he had to be supported to the scale with cold compresses on his neck because of faintness.

That a 10-year-old child should be given a prescription drug that can cause heart failure, disturbances of the heart rate and rhythm, kidney problems, even death when used inappropriately is sad and scary but what makes it worse is that he took Lasix with the knowledge of the athletic director of his football league! Moreover, the adult director said he recommends the prescription drug to several boys each year so they can "make weight" and play on the team of their choice. If the parents can't obtain the drug, he helps them get it.

"I personally see nothing wrong," he told the *Tribune*. "I do not condone more than one (tablet), and only three hours before a weigh-in, which is a lot safer than putting a finger down his throat, or taking an enema, or sitting in a sauna for three or four days, or wrapping up in plastic, or not eating at all." Of course, none of those practices is acceptable. The youth was taken to his pediatrician after the incident. When the doctor heard the tale, he called the police. The coach protested: "If it's not abused, it's 100 times safer than what some of these high school kids are taking."

This tale illustrates everything that is wrong with the American attitude toward sports. The wrong messages being sent are that it's OK to cheat to gain a sports advantage and that using chemicals to alter your body to play sports is OK. No youngster should seriously risk his health playing any sport. No youngster should be shown by example that his coach and/or parents think that cheating is OK. With this type of message, it is not unreasonable to assume that today it may be a diuretic and tomorrow a steroid or whatever else will confer a winning edge. So long as unethical behavior in the service of sport is accepted, we will continue to have both a cheating problem and a drug problem of massive proportions.

---

make sports contests fair and to encourage young athletes to be good sportsmen is because their ethical conduct on the playing field lays a foundation for later ethical conduct in life. Life is a team sport. Competitiveness and a fierce desire to win are qualities that have made this nation great. But before we allow our children to compete, we must first establish in them a moral and ethical foundation so they have boundaries they will not cross in pursuit of victory.

"Show me a good and gracious loser and I'll show you a failure," said Notre Dame's legendary football coach Knute Rockne, but children need to learn how to do their best, how to win, and how to lose. Sadly, youngsters who participate in sports, particularly those with athletic ability, often find themselves enmeshed in highly stressful situations early in life when they should still be learning what it takes to be a decent person. There are examples in every sport of young athletes who drop out because they were pushed too fast. They end up with psychic burnout or develop overuse injuries at a young age. Other young athletes may be tempted to resort to drugs. When children are inculcated with a "winning is the *only* thing" attitude, performance-enhancing drug use and other forms of cheating become very rational behavior.

When youth sports stops being about skills development and being part of a team effort and starts being consumed with winning, kids learn another lesson. They become afraid of losing, and too many of them grow up afraid to take chances because they might not be successful. The incomparable Michael Jordan has said he doesn't fear losing; it is "not trying" that he can't accept. If kids grow up wanting to "be like Mike," let us hope they try to emulate his attitude as much as his basketball skills.

SOCIETAL ATTITUDES AND NATIONAL PRIDE

If we decide that the use of performance-enhancing drugs may cause fundamental changes in the nature of sports that are not acceptable, the question then becomes: Can we change societal attitudes? Health educators have made some inroads in changing several high-risk behaviors, such as high-fat diets, sedentary lifestyles, and smoking. They have been able to do this, in part, because a wealth of scientific data exists that correlates habits and health risks. Some individuals have made lifestyle changes because the attitudes of society toward health risks has changed, and now there is public disapproval of some risky behaviors. Drunk driving and smoking have been altered by changed attitudes in society.

Turning to sports, the first obvious difference is that anabolic steroids don't usually cause athletes to behave in ways that bring public disapproval. They often demonstrate improvements in physical performance and appearance. Society is much less likely to shun these people. In fact, the adulation of fans, the media, and peers serves as a strong reinforcement, as do the financial, material, and sexual rewards that come with athletic success.

When it comes to international sports, there is an added element of national pride. For several years before the 1996 Olympic Games, there was great concern about the Chinese female athletes who would be coming to Atlanta. Press coverage had focused attention on the exploits of the Chinese women and stimulated public concern about whether a fair contest would be possible. A 1995 *Sports Illustrated* article noted that Chinese distance runners were doing an incredible volume of training. Women ran almost a marathon a day at higher altitudes, and then followed that up with sprint training. This type of training schedule flies in the face of stress studies that

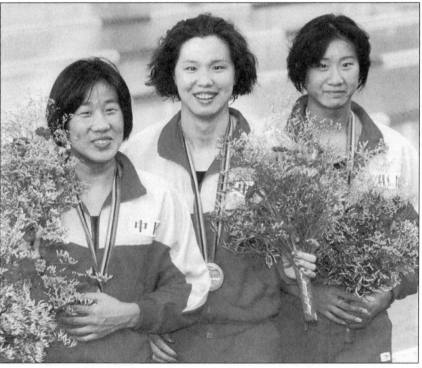

Suspicions surrounding the possible drug use by the Chinese women's swim team, shown here, has continued to surface despite their coaches' claims that their world record-breaking performances result from superior, more intense training schedules.

have demonstrated that humans don't have enough adaptive energy to do both.

The story in swimming was much the same. FINA, the international sports governing body for swimming, keeps track of the top 25 times recorded each year for each of the recognized events in swimming. When FINA issued the 1992 top 25 rankings, only 28 Chinese women made the list of 325. In 1993, the Chinese women had 101 top 25 rankings out of a total of 325. This is an enormous change over a very short period of time. The fact that China has only eight male swimmers who achieved top 25 rankings raises the index of suspicion about drug use even more because women make proportionally greater gains on steroids. It began to sound far too much like the East German story where the female swimmers came from nowhere in the 1970s and then dominated women's swimming for a decade. After the Berlin Wall fell, the world learned that sophisticated treatment with steroids and other drugs was the foundation of the East German success.

The Chinese women did not dominate in Atlanta, however. Drug testing at the Asian Games preceding the 1996 Olympics caught some Chinese female athletes who were using steroids. Some of these women have since dropped from public view in their sports. It is unlikely the story of why the Chinese female athletes receded from their dominant position before the Games will ever be known, but public opinion may have played a part. The Chinese may be regrouping to come back in force in the 2000 Olympic Games. Communist China, at least in the recent past, obviously intends to use international athletics as a means to showcase its society. Because China is a closed society, and the State controls the pharmaceutical industry, they have the motive and opportunity to develop designer drugs and perfect other strategies to subvert drug testing.

ALTERNATIVES FOR ACTION

What are the alternatives for dealing with steroids and other performance-enhancing drugs? They include legalization, legislation and enforcement, education, and/or changing societal values and attitudes about physical appearance and winning in sports. The first, legalizing drugs, would force virtually all athletes to become drug users if they wanted to be competitive, and it would reinforce the notion that any action in the service of winning is OK. That alternative is clearly unacceptable. Some people contend, however, that athletes in certain sports are already faced with the dilemma of using drugs or accepting that they cannot be truly competitive.

An alternative solution is to deny that a serious problem exists. Many sports fans are currently embracing this alternative because it does not conflict with a fixation on winning and appearance. The formula for this alternative is fairly simple. First, turn a blind eye to obvious signs of drug use like athletes of superhuman size, strength, or speed. Next, publicly proclaim victory over the problem because drug testing exists, even though it has many obvious loopholes. Finally, hang an anti-steroid poster in the school weight room and schedule the annual showing of a video depicting the evils of steroids.

It takes courage to abandon this highly seductive strategy of denial, but if we do, real progress is possible. At the close of the Steroid Congress in Prague, 12 recommendations were issued that offer some hope for developing alternative strategies for dealing with steroids if they can be implemented:

- Further research on public health and social consequences should be encouraged.
- Governments and international organizations should share information.
- National and international laboratories should consider collecting and sharing reference standards and analytical methodologies.
- Health, police, customs, and policy officials involved in the issues of drug control, abuse, and trafficking should familiarize themselves with the available information on steroids.
- Prevention efforts should be strengthened.
- Both governments and sports bodies should enhance their progress in detecting the use of anabolic steroids.
- Legislation should be looked at with a view to strengthening controls over anabolic steroids.
- National regulatory authorities and sports organizations should cooperate in developing a joint strategy to combat the abuse of anabolic steroids.
- National authorities should consider increasing cooperation on international commerce of anabolic agents.

- Police and customs authorities should provide operational assistance to each other in the investigation of trafficking in anabolic steroids.
- The ICPO/Interpol and Customs Cooperation Council should continue to collect, review, and analyze existing information so as to assist in developing programs on anabolic steroid abuse and trafficking.
- The World Health Organization should continue its analysis of global trends regarding the use and abuse of anabolic agents and its assessment of current educational, prevention, and regulatory activities.

Will any of these recommendations, if implemented, change the level of drug use at the professional and Olympic levels? Probably not. There is simply too much money at stake, and many of the drugs work too well to think otherwise. The health and spiritual well-being of our children are so vital that we can ill afford to throw up our hands in despair. The avenue that appears to offer the most promise with our children is education. The prevention program developed by Dr. Linn Goldberg and the group at the Oregon Health Sciences University works (see Chapter 6). That model requires a concerted community effort, but it is effective.

Beyond education, we are left with the struggle to change the values of society. Whether it is possible to change an unhealthy preoccupation with winning at any cost remains to be seen. Far too many of us focus on the individual rewards of athletic success but fail to realize that professional sports careers are only a dream for all but a very few people. For example, even with 30 teams in the National Football League, there is room for less than 1,500 players. The probability of a high school athlete collecting a paycheck in the NBA or NFL is about 1/10,000.

In tennis, there are hundreds of professionals, but only a few receive appearance fees and tournament winnings. The same is true in golf and other professional sports. Only a handful of Olympic athletes are ever able to capitalize on their sports success. Clearly, preparing for a career in professional sports is risky business because it requires focusing on getting a job that, statistically, doesn't exist. The available data indicate that misguided parents and coaches help perpetuate the idea of the "Rocky" story when the reality is that they have almost as good a chance to win the lottery as to guide a child into professional sports. Moreover, this attitude sends an unspoken message that participating in sports is not worth anything unless the participant can parlay that into a paying job.

There are those who argue that our attitudes and values related to sports and appearance are too deeply entrenched to change, and that may be true. If it is, we must resign ourselves to the prospect of children and teens using dangerous drugs with known short-term and unknown long-term negative health consequences. It certainly is true that no amount of legislation or drug testing will work unless society does decide that its fixation with winning and appearance is unhealthy. But the individual and societal rewards of changing our attitudes and making sports competition a healthy activity make the goal worth the pursuit.

SUGGESTED READINGS

Bamberger, M., and D. Yaeger. 1997. Over the edge. *Sports Illustrated,* 14 April, 62-70.

Bissinger, H.G. (1990). *Friday Night Lights.* Addison-Wesley Publishing Company, Inc., N.Y.

Buckley et al. (1988). Estimated prevalence of anabolic steroid use among male hughh school seniors. *Journal of the American Medical Association.*

Clark, N. 1997. *Nancy Clark's sports nutrition guidebook (2nd ed.).* Champaign, IL: Human Kinetics.

Courson, S., and Schreiber, L. 1991. *False glory.* Stamford, CT: Longmeadow Press.

Dubin, C. 1990. *Commission of inquiry into the use of drugs and banned practices intended to increase athletic performance.* Ottawa, Ontario, Canada: Canadian Government Publishing Centre.

Fleck, S. J., and W. J. Kraemer. 1997. *Designing resistance training programs (2nd ed.).* Champaign, IL: Human Kinetics.

Fleck, S. J., and W. J. Kraemer. 1996. *Periodization breakthrough!* New York: Advanced Research Press.

Francis, C. 1990. *Speed trap.* New York: St. Martin's Press.

Franke, W., and B. Berendonk. 1997. Hormonal doping and androgenization of athletes: A secret program of the German Democratic Republic government. *Clinical Chemistry,* 43:7, 1262-1279.

Goldberg, L. and D. L. Elliot. 1994. *Exercise for Prevention and Treatment of Illness.* F.A. Davis, Philadelphia.

Hoberman, J. 1992. *Mortal engines.* New York: Free Press.

Kraemer, W. J., and S. J. Fleck. 1993. *Strength training for young athletes.* Champaign, IL.: Human Kinetics.

Lucas, J. 1992. *Future of the Olympic Games.* Champaign, IL: Human Kinetics.

Voy, R. 1991. *Drugs, sport, and politics.* Champaign, IL: Human Kinetics.

Yesalis, C. E., ed. 1993. *Anabolic steroids in sport and exercise.* Champaign, IL: Human Kinetics.

Yesalis, C., et al. 1993. Anabolic-androgenic steroid use in the United States. *Journal of the American Medical Association.* 270:10, 1217-1221.

INDEX

ABOUT THE AUTHORS

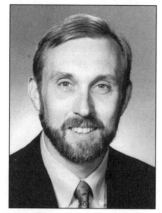
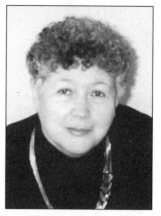

Dr. Charles Yesalis   Virginia S. Cowart

Dr. Charles Yesalis received his Bachelor of Science and Master of Public Health degrees from the University of Michigan, and he was awarded his doctoral degree from Johns Hopkins School of Hygiene and Public Health in 1975. He then joined the faculty at Johns Hopkins for one year. From 1976 to 1986, Yesalis was a member of the Department of Preventive Medicine and Environmental Health at the University of Iowa. He is currently a professor of health policy and administration and exercise and sport science at The Pennsylvania State University.

Since 1980, much of Dr. Yesalis' research has been devoted to the nonmedical use of anabolic steroids and other performance enhancing drugs. In 1988 he directed the first national study of steroid use among adolescents and was the first to present evidence of psychological dependence on the drug. In a 1993 nationwide survey, Yesalis and his colleagues were the first to present an estimate of steroid use in the U.S. population and demonstrate an association between anabolic steroid use and violent behavior and the use of other illicit drugs and alcohol. That same year he edited the book, *Anabolic Steroids in Sport and Exercise*.

On three occasions Yesalis has been asked to testify before the U.S. Congress on legislation related to the control of anabolic steroids and growth hormone abuse. He also has been a consultant to the U.S. Senate Judiciary Committee, the Drug Enforcement Administration, the Federal Bureau of Investigation, the American Medical Association, the NFL Players Association, the U.S. Olympic Committee, the National Collegiate Athletic Association, and the National Strength and Conditioning Association.

Virginia S. Cowart is a Chicago-based medical writer who has been writing about anabolic steroids for more than a decade. Her series on drugs and sport written for the Journal of the American Medical Association (JAMA) was one of the first detailed reports on the scientific response to increased drug use among athletes. She is also the coauthor of *Anabolic Steroids/Altered States*, which was written in 1990 with Dr. James Wright.

A graduate of the University of Kentucky, Cowart has held the position of associate editor of the medical news section of JAMA and science editor for the University of Chicago Office of Public Information. She has been a contributor to many sports medicine publications, and she wrote the original entry on steroids for *Encyclopedia Britannica*.

ALSO AVAILABLE FROM HUMAN KINETICS

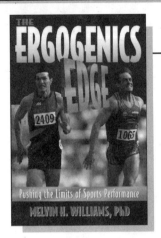

Help maximize your athletic potential by going beyond traditional sports conditioning while staying within the rules. Dr. Mel Williams presents nearly every current nutritional, pharmacological, physiological, biomechanical, and psychological means used to aid sports performance.

1997 • Paper • 328 pp • Item PWIL0545
ISBN 0-88011-545-9 • $17.95 ($26.95 Canadian)

Power Eating provides no-nonsense advice on eating to increase your muscle strength and power; answers to commons sports nutrition questions; complete breakdowns of carbohydrate, protein, fat, and total calories for recommended foods; and eight sample diet plans.

1998 • Paper • 240 pp • Item PKLE0702
ISBN 0-088011-702-8 • $15.95 ($23.95 Canadian)

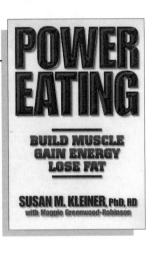

Written by leading experts in steroid research and clinical sports medicine, this book helps dispel common myths and provides you with complete facts about anabolic steroids in sport and exercise.

1993 • Cloth • 360 pp • Item BYES0401
ISBN 0-87322-401-9 • $38.00 ($56.95 Canadian)

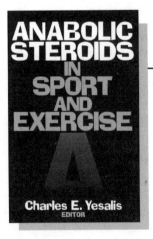

HUMAN KINETICS
The Premier Publisher for Sports & Fitness
http://www.humankinetics.com/
2335

For more information or to place your order, U.S. customers call toll-free 1-800-747-4457. Customers outside the U.S. use the appropriate telephone number/address shown in the front of this book.